THE
ASPERGER'S
Answer Book

The Top 300 Questions Parents Ask

SUSAN ASHLEY, PH.D.

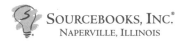
SOURCEBOOKS, INC.®
NAPERVILLE, ILLINOIS

Published by Sourcebooks, Inc.
P.O. Box 4410, Naperville, Illinois 60567-4410
(630) 961-3900
Fax: (630) 961-2168
www.sourcebooks.com

Library of Congress Cataloging-in-Publication Data

Ashley, Susan, PhD.
  The Asperger's answer book : the top 300 questions parents ask / Susan Ashley.
       p. cm.
  Includes bibliographical references and index.
  ISBN-13: 978-1-4022-0807-2
  ISBN-10: 1-4022-0807-3
  1. Asperger's syndrome in children--Popular works. I. Title.

RJ506.A9A77 2006
618.92'858832--dc22

2006020833

Printed and bound in the United States of America.
CH 10 9 8 7 6 5 4 3 2

Dedication

For today's child and tomorrow's adult

Acknowledgments

The writing of this book would never have been possible without the many children with Asperger's Disorder whom I have had the great fortune to meet and share their lives. While a child psychologist learns from workshops, seminars, and books, it is the time spent with these children that has been the greatest teacher to me in my journey with Asperger's Disorder. I have felt honored by the parents who selected me to be their child's psychologist. While it has been my pleasure to help these children, it has been my personal joy to know each and every one.

The words "thank you" do not capture the depth of my gratitude to my research assistant Tiffany Kleoni Witwit. It is only with her help that this book is able to provide the solid research-based findings

A word of gratitude for Ed Brostoff, MA, special education advocate, for sharing his knowledge of special education.

Many thanks to Doreen Granpeesheh, PhD, BC, BA, founder and director of the Center for Autism and Related Disorders in Tarzana, CA, for her expertise on autism.

Appreciation goes to my copy editors Tara VanTimmeren and Rachel Jay who ensure that I have put the commas, colons, and periods in all the right places, and to Katie Olsen for her attention to detail throughout the production of this book.

Once again it was my great pleasure to work with Senior Editor Bethany Brown. She has a passion for child psychology and Asperger's Disorder that is the inspiration that gave life to this book.

To Teri for her never-ending supply of enthusiasm for whatever endeavor I pursue, including this book.

As always, my deepest appreciation to Stan for everything, and more.

Contents

Introduction

The world of Asperger's Disorder is confusing and overwhelming. From the moment you suspect your child has Asperger's Disorder, also known as Asperger's Syndrome, you begin a journey that seems to have no road map. Once your child is diagnosed, the destination becomes even less clear.

- Is it Asperger's Disorder or high-functioning autism?
- Will your child be able to make friends?
- What about special education?
- Does your child need to be tested?
- How can your child learn social skills?

The list of questions goes on and on, but the answers are difficult to find.

The Asperger's Answer Book gives you the answers to your most important questions. Over sixteen years in private practice has given me the inside perspective of what parents really want to know. The answers in this book are the same answers I would give to you if we were having a face-to-face consultation in my office. The answers are based on the current research and state-of-the-art psychological techniques.

This book differs from all other books about Asperger's Disorder because, like a dictionary, this book can be used as a reference. Over the years, as your child progresses through the various stages of this disorder, you will have *The Asperger's Answer Book* on your reference shelf to find the answers to your new questions.

The Asperger's Answer Book will transform you into a well-informed parent. You will have extensive knowledge direct from a child psychologist who treats Asperger's Disorder. You will have straight-forward, no-holds-barred, honest information about what you are likely to face over the years in raising your child with Asperger's Disorder. You will have the most current information based on research and clinical practice.

In writing *The Asperger's Answer Book*, it is my hope that it becomes your guidebook and that you will use it frequently. I hope that you will turn to this book each time you have a question. It is my wish that you will use the numerous techniques in this book that I, and many other child psychologists, have used over the years in treating children with Asperger's Disorder. I hope that you find the inspiration to apply the techniques despite the tireless effort it requires on your part. While some of your reward for your hard work will come in the days, weeks, and months ahead, your true reward will come in the years ahead when you see your child suc-ceed in school, find his place with friends, like who he has become, and find a passion that he can make his life's work.

Chapter 1

THE ABCs OF ASPERGER'S DISORDER

- What is Asperger's Disorder?
- What are the social interaction symptoms of Asperger's Disorder?
- What are the thinking problems seen in Asperger's Disorder?
- What are the emotional problems seen in Asperger's Disorder?
- What are the intense preoccupations seen in Asperger's Disorder?
- What are the repetitive behaviors, routines, and movements seen in Asperger's Disorder?
- What are the play problems seen in Asperger's Disorder?
- What are the speech and language problems seen in Asperger's Disorder?
- What are the motor skills problems seen in Asperger's Disorder?
- What are the sensitivity problems seen in Asperger's Disorder?
- What does the Asperger's Disorder child look like in daily life?
- What does the preschool child with Asperger's Disorder look like?
- What does the elementary child with Asperger's Disorder look like?
- What does the adolescent with Asperger's Disorder look like?
- How is Asperger's Disorder different from autism?
- How is Asperger's Disorder different from high-functioning autism?
- How common is Asperger's Disorder?
- Is Asperger's Disorder a real disorder?
- Is Asperger's Disorder caused by something in the brain?
- Is Asperger's Disorder genetic?
- What other factors are suspected of causing Asperger's Disorder?
- Is there a cure for Asperger's Disorder?
- How is Asperger's Disorder treated?
- Can medication help Asperger's Disorder?

What is Asperger's Disorder?

Asperger's Disorder, which will be referred to as AD throughout this book, is considered a pervasive developmental disorder. This means it causes significant problems in many areas of the child's development, including socialization, communication, behavior, thinking, and activities.

Children, teens, and adults who have AD have significant problems with:

1. Socializing with others
2. Thinking
3. Emotions
4. Intense preoccupation with one or two topics
5. Repetitive routines, behaviors, and movements
6. Play
7. Speech and language
8. Motor skills
9. Sensitivity to sensations of sound, light, or touch

Individuals with AD are different from people with other pervasive developmental disorders in that they do not have significant delays in language, cognitive development, or self-help skills.

Symptoms of AD are seen in every setting, including at home, in the classroom, on the playground, and in after-school and extracurricular activities. Virtually every area of the AD child's life is affected.

Symptoms of AD may begin to develop as early as age two; however, it is most often recognized after the child starts school, where his unusual manner of talking and failure to play appropriately with his peers begins to surface. The combination of symptoms results in a child who is identified by others as "odd" and is quickly rejected by his peers.

Symptoms of AD
Social
- Often prefers to be by himself
- Unaware of how his behavior and/or comments affect others
- Seems uninterested in activities that involve competition
- Does not seem influenced by peer pressure, fads, trends, or pop culture
- Inability to interact with peers
- Lack of desire to interact with peers
- Poor appreciation of social cues and body language
- Limited facial expressions
- Socially inappropriate responses
- Seems uninterested in what others have to say in a conversation
- Does not ask others questions or their opinions
- Makes limited eye contact
- Limited use of expressive hand or body gestures
- Does not look others in the eye

Thinking Patterns
- Impressive long-term memory for facts
- Seems almost obsessed with a particular topic
- Expects others to understand what he thinks without telling them
- Does not ask for clarification when confused
- Cannot imagine what others are thinking
- Cannot interpret other's intentions

Emotions
- Does not understand how other people feel; lacks empathy
- Extreme reactions to minor upsets
- Fails to modify emotional expression to match the situation
- Feelings are all-or-none
- Cannot read emotions of people's faces

Intense Preoccupation with One or Two Topics
- Fanatical about his interest
- Seems obsessed with interest
- Talks incessantly about his interest
- Little interest in other topics
- Pursues advanced knowledge about his interest
- Shows off knowledge in almost encyclopedic manner

Repetitive Routines, Behaviors, and Movements
- Sticks to rigid routine
- Difficulty being flexible
- Imposes routine on others
- Needs excessive reassurance when changes take place
- Upset by changes in routine
- Repetitive, senseless body movements

Play
- Seems to not understand how to play with other children
- Does not know unspoken rules of play
- Often prefers to play by himself rather than with peers
- Uses playmates as objects
- Intense reaction if play does not go his way
- Controlling of playmates
- Difficulty sharing toys
- Lacks imaginative play

Speech and Language
- Interprets things literally
- Does not understand figures of speech, metaphors
- Has an unusual tone of voice
- Talks in an overly precise manner
- Uses advanced vocabulary
- Odd rhythm
- Peculiar voice characteristics

Motor Skills
- Poor coordination
- Poor ball play
- Odd gait when walking or running
- Poor writing

Sensory Sensitivity
- Overly reactive to sounds
- Overly reactive to lights
- Overly reactive to fabrics
- Resistant to food textures

What are the social interaction symptoms of Asperger's Disorder?

Children with AD have a variety of symptoms that prevent them from making and sustaining friendships. Each time we talk, play, or interact with another person, there is an unspoken understanding that we both intuitively understand the rules of interacting. We know that we should look one another in the eye, listen and respond to what the other person has to say, stick to the conversation, take turns, and share in the other person's excitement. The child with AD, however, does not know what the rules are and, even when repeatedly taught them, has little or no interest in following them and does not understand their purpose.

The AD child does not:

- Engage in normal eye contact
- Show much interest in other people
- Display empathy for other people
- Share in the interests and achievements of others
- Understand body language
- Converse on topic
- Respond to what others are saying
- Read social cues

The AD child is not on the same social page as others. He is highly self-focused and has little interest in others. He seems blind to the idea that others have thoughts, feelings, and interests that they too want to share.

What are the thinking problems seen in Asperger's Disorder?

Much of the difficulty AD children and teens have stems from their problems in thinking. Despite the vast majority of those with AD having average to above average intelligence, all have significant thinking problems. They are excellent in thinking about things but extremely poor in thinking about people. They have an inability to understand what is going on in the minds of others. They lack empathy and are unable to understand how other people feel and how they might react to their words and behavior. Thinking problems seen in AD include:

- Unaware of other's feelings
- Inability to read other people's intentions
- Viewing things in black-and-white
- Inability to see another person's perspective
- Rigid adherence to rules
- Inability to tell what others are thinking
- Perfectionistic thinking
- Interpreting others' words literally
- Catastrophic thinking
- Rigid thinking
- Perseverative thinking
- Failure to generalize

What are the emotional problems seen in Asperger's Disorder?

The AD child has difficulties with emotions in several ways. She has difficulty understanding emotions and controlling how she expresses her feelings, and does not understand how other people feel.

Difficulty with emotions includes:
- Difficulty reading facial expressions
- Limited use of facial expressions
- Lack of empathy
- Blind to the feelings of others

The AD child seems to move through life as if she is the only one who has feelings.

Her emotion at any given time is what matters to her, regardless of what is happening around her. It is not that she is purposely uncaring, callous, or coldhearted; she simply cannot walk in another person's emotional shoes. If a peer is talking about the death of his pet over the weekend, the AD child will interrupt to talk about her visit to the airplane show. The AD child cannot understand why she should let the other boy talk about his grief and forgo her talk about the airplane show. She will interrupt, show obvious signs of being impatient, and repeatedly ask if it is her turn yet. This type of self-centeredness, lack of empathy, and selfishness works quickly to get her rejected as a friend.

What are the intense preoccupations seen in Asperger's Disorder?

While most children have a favorite toy, area of interest, or object they like to collect, they also are very curious, interested, and excited about a wide variety of things. The AD child is not. He typically has one area that he is interested in, and the rest of the world holds little curiosity for him. Once the AD child develops an affinity for a particular subject or object, he becomes preoccupied—some parents would even say obsessed.

Dinosaurs, trains, and airplanes are common areas of interest. Many a child is fascinated with dinosaurs and learns their names and collects the toy figurines. The AD child, however, goes overboard and has a sole focus of gaining extensive, almost expert knowledge and vocabulary.

What separates the AD child from the other children who collect dinosaurs is his exclusive focus on dinosaurs. Every conversation becomes focused on his dinosaur knowledge, whether or not others want to hear about it. He talks literally nonstop, never pausing for a second and never giving the other person a chance to join in, change the subject, or even say he must leave.

What are the repetitive routines, behaviors, and movements seen in Asperger's Disorder?

Children with AD typically prefer routine and can become quite irritable if things do not go as expected. Anxiety is reduced when they have the sense of control that comes with knowing what is going to happen. Minor changes that seem meaningless to others can result in intense reactions for children with AD, who have little ability to adapt to unexpected changes and recover from the upset they feel if things did not go as planned. Tantrums, refusal to cooperate, and aggression can occur for some AD children who cannot handle changes.

Children with AD may also have set behaviors that they "must" do. Oftentimes these behaviors make no sense to others and serve no purpose. The AD child may have to walk down the hall on a certain side or have to touch a chair with his index finger. Attempts to prevent him from doing the behaviors can result in anger, tears, or tantrums.

Movements can be senseless and odd. They may use odd hand gestures repetitively or engage in rocking of their body. These behaviors are generally not thought of as problematic unless they are harmful or causing significant disruption in behavior or teasing by peers.

What are the play problems seen in Asperger's Disorder?

Play comes naturally to children. When first playing with other children their age, babies and toddlers play alongside one another. As they move from toddler to kindergarten years, they begin to play cooperatively together with the same theme and purpose. Although it is common for children to want to be the one in charge of the play, they somehow figure out how to play with their peers and get along by making compromises. AD children do not figure this out. While they are interested in playing with their peers, they are more interested in using their playmate for their own purpose rather than to have a mutually rewarding play experience.

Play problems of the AD child include:
- Limited cooperative play
- Narrow range of play interests
- Highly repetitive play behaviors
- Limited imaginative play
- Dominating the play

More than simply being bossy, the AD child uses her playmate almost as another toy, something she can direct and maneuver to her liking. She has no interest in the fun of actually being with her peer and playing "together." If her peer does not play exactly how she wants him to, the fun is ruined.

What are the speech and language problems seen in AD?

Individuals with AD may start to speak later than normally expected but eventually catch up to their peers. If speech is delayed, no serious problems remain; however, the AD child does speak in an unusual manner. He can express his thoughts just fine but tends to sound odd in a variety of ways, including:

- Repeated questioning
- Lecturing others in a monologue instead of conversing
- Using an advanced vocabulary
- Overly precise way of saying words
- Adultlike way of talking
- Odd tone of voice
- Dominating conversations with favorite topic
- Endless talking
- Failure to ask for an explanation when confused
- Voice lacks emotion

Upon meeting a child with AD, one quickly hears an odd tone of voice that may sound mechanical and robotic, as if there were no feelings behind the words. His manner of speaking may not be obvious to others as a symptom of a disorder. More often others simply find the AD child a poor choice for conversation.

What are the motor skills problems seen in AD?

Motor skills represent a person's ability to move their body in big ways, such as running, jumping, or throwing a ball, and move their body in small ways such as writing, buttoning, and using a safety pin. Big body movements are called "gross motor" skills while the smaller movements with the hands are called "fine motor" skills. Both types of movements can be difficult for children with AD. Typically AD children are slow to develop their motor skills and lag behind their peers.

Typical motor skill problems of AD include:

- Clumsiness
- Poor ball play
- Difficulty imitating body movements
- Weak hand-eye coordination
- Trouble balancing on one leg

While one can certainly get through life without being good at balancing on one leg, physical play is one of the main ways children interact with each other. Those who cannot catch or throw a ball are not selected for ball games. Clumsy children who accidentally knock over game pieces or towers of blocks are a source of irritation to peers. Classmates are easily upset when the AD child drops the ball, strikes out, or misses the hoop. Repeated public failure in physical play contributes to teasing and social rejection.

What are the sensitivity problems in AD?

While not all children with AD are overly reactive to stimulation, there are many who show extreme sensitivity. They can be excessively sensitive to sound, touch, and light. Noises that others hardly notice can be very irritating to the AD child, and they lack the ability to screen it out or get used to it. Sudden loud noises are particularly upsetting, as are background noises that most others are not aware of. Bright lights and fluorescent lights can be bothersome. Many AD children are particularly picky about the clothing they wear. Some are able to tell their parents that the seam at the toe of the sock is bothersome to them, and the parent can begin the hunt for seamless socks. Others, however, are not able to identify the cause of the irritation and express it in the form of an angry outburst or tantrum that appears to come from nowhere. AD children can also have sensitivities to the textures of various foods and refuse to eat whole categories of foods.

Some children will have one or two very specific sensitivities while others have so many that it is almost impossible for their parent to control the environment to try to prevent the offending stimulus.

What does the Asperger's Disorder child look like in daily life?

AD children and teens are average or bright intellectually, but they are perceived by others to be odd socially. They are self-focused and show little awareness or interest in others except for having an audience to talk to about their very specific and narrow interests. The AD child talks to and lectures rather than conversing with others. He does not like to listen, and once others are done talking, he does not respond to what they said but restarts where he left off in his monologue.

AD children have trouble with eye contact, body language, and the give and take of conversations and relationships. Often extremely interested in one or two subjects, they will focus most of their energy and conversation around that topic. They do not understand how to behave towards others; they miss out on nonverbal cues because they do not understand facial expressions, gestures, and body language. They fail to consider what others might need and instead focus on their own thoughts, feelings, and desires. They dominate conversations and become frustrated when others interrupt or try to change the subject. They cannot shift gears in conversations or activities without upset.

What does the preschool child with AD look like?

Toddlers with AD may seem normal in the home. However, once they enter preschool, symptoms of AD begin to surface when they fail to initiate play with their peers and seem content to be "in their own world." They interact better with their teachers than their peers. Odd behaviors of being silly, loud, aggressive, or socially withdrawn are frequently seen in preschool. Hyperactivity, inattention, and emotional outbursts are not surprising and can make distinguishing between AD and Attention Deficit Hyperactivity Disorder (ADHD) difficult.

Transitioning from one activity to another often results in difficulties. Repetitive motor movements may be seen as well. You may observe her excellent memory skills, with the child able to recite dialogue from favorite cartoons and movies. Enthusiasm for collecting certain toys or objects is often seen. Even at this young age, the focus of the collection is more on organizing, counting, or moving the objects rather than playing with them. Accelerated language development is generally seen and young AD children often impress adults as remarkably verbal, bright, and adultlike in the way they speak. However, they simultaneously have trouble with keeping the volume of their voice appropriate for the situation and having a conversation where the other person can participate, and they fail to use gestures when talking.

What does the elementary child with AD look like?

The early signs of social skills problems possibly present during preschool become very apparent in elementary school. The AD child will generally be either withdrawn from social interactions, preferring to stay by himself, or quite the opposite: he is intrusive, loud, relentless, and annoying to his peers. AD children's inability to understand social behavior can result in aggression when they misinterpret other children's behavior as purposely "out to get them," and they retaliate with hitting or other outbursts of violence.

Sadly, their unusual manner of interacting is obvious and their peers quickly learn to avoid them. By mid-elementary school, the AD child is aware that he is not fitting in, but does not understand why.

Their typically advanced intellect and reading and vocabulary skills can make it confusing for the teacher to understand how a child so smart can exhibit such immature behavior. Teachers may experience trouble getting the AD child to become engaged in activities other than his interest. Outbursts of talking back, refusal to comply, and tantrums occur in some AD children who have particular difficulty with transitioning between classroom activities. However, not all AD children have behavior problems, and their difficulties may be limited to the social arena.

What does the adolescent with Asperger's Disorder look like?

The social arena continues to cause the greatest difficulty for the adolescent with AD. In the teenage years, friendships become of primary importance and those who do not fit in are often teased and rejected, making them vulnerable to depression. Middle school has a tremendous amount of peer pressure to be "cool" and to be just like everyone else. This is hard on many children, but in particular for AD children, who lack the skills to try to fit in. While others their age make friendships that involve trust, secrets, and common interests, the AD teen does not have friends and begins to identify that his differences are responsible for why he is lonely.

Social life may improve in high school as there is less pressure to be just like everyone else. At this age, teens form their individual identities, and they view differences in a less negative light than in middle school. High school usually offers more opportunities for finding a group to belong to. Being labeled a "computer nerd" or "bookworm" is no longer viewed as so negative and the AD child will likely find others with similar interests to socialize with.

How is Asperger's Disorder different from autism?

Formally called Autistic Disorder, autism, like AD, is a pervasive developmental disorder. The symptoms of autism include markedly abnormal social interaction and communication, and a restricted range of activities and interests. These are the same symptoms as AD, so how are the two disorders different?

Signs of autism start far earlier than those of AD and allow for diagnosis to be made usually by age two to two and a half. In contrast, the symptoms of AD are less apparent, noticed at the earliest in preschool. More often, however, it is not until mid-elementary school years that children with AD are diagnosed. Estimates are 10 percent of those with AD receive their diagnosis at age four, 50 percent between ages five and ten, 20 percent between ages ten and twelve, and the remaining 20 percent after the onset of adolescence.

Many researchers and mental health professionals hold the view that AD and autism are two distinct disorders. Currently, the more widely held view is that AD is probably a high-functioning form of autism. The trend is to view both disorders as being on a continuum from very low-functioning to very high-functioning. This continuum is referred to as Autism Spectrum Disorders or ASD. Those on the low end of the spectrum are diagnosed with Autistic Disorder due to their very severe symptoms; they function quite poorly in most areas of life and many fail to achieve independent adult functioning. Those on the high end of the spectrum are considered to have AD with mild symptoms; they function relatively well with an eventual outcome of independence in adulthood. The difference between Autistic Disorder and AD is quite clear and easy for even non-professionals to see. The difficulty comes in distinguishing between very high-functioning autism (HFA) and AD.

How is Asperger's Disorder different from high-functioning autism?

High-functioning autism (HFA) is not a formal diagnosis but a term many doctors, teachers, and researchers use. This group functions at a very high level, as do children with AD, but they also have some symptoms consistent with autism. Where to draw the line between HFA and AD is not at all clear, and no criteria exist to distinguish between the two. Some professionals believe they are one and the same, so the term HFA should be eliminated. Others, however, see AD as simply a very high level of autism.

The language used to label these disorders can be incredibly confusing. You may be told your child has autism, a high-functioning form of autism on the autism spectrum called Asperger's. How do you tell which it is, and does it really matter?

The difference between autism and AD matters a lot. Prognosis, school placement, and services available are very different for autism than AD. Materials that you read, techniques you use for parenting, and support groups you will become involved in all differ substantially as well.

However, distinctions between HFA and AD may be less important. Provided your child is getting the proper services to address his symptoms, the exact label has less meaning. It is important that those working with your child follow the philosophy of "treat the child, not the diagnosis."

Comparison of Autism and Asperger's

This chart highlights some of the differences in the major symptoms of autism and Asperger's. The severities of symptoms presented are general descriptions and are not for purposes of diagnosis. Each child is unique and will likely have a range of functioning in these areas.

Comparison of Autism and Asperger's

Symptom	Severe Autism	Moderate Autism	Mild Autism	Asperger's Disorder
Socialization	Indifferent, disinterested in others	Seeks others for physical needs	Accepts if approached by others	Seeks others for one-sided interaction
Communication	Uses negative behavior to communicate	Uses gestures to communicate	Responds if approached by others	Seeks others for one-sided talking
Language	None or echolalia—repeats what others say	Echolalia and some language to communicate	Poor pragmatics, odd use of pronouns and words	Very good, repetitive, literal, excessive, odd
Peer Play	No	No	Parallel play but poor interaction	Seeks others for one-sided play
Sensory Sensitivity	Varies, severe to none	Varies, significant to none	Varies, none to moderate or mild	Varies, none to moderate or mild

Imaginative Play	None	Copies others	Repetitive play, little imaginative	Repetitive play, limited imaginative play
Repetitive Activities	Senseless body movements, may be self-injurious	Repeated body movements and touching objects	Rituals with objects or body movements	Talking, questioning; may have some body movements, some rituals
Reaction to Change	Insists on sameness, extreme reaction	Insists on sameness, severe to moderate reaction	Insists on sameness, moderate reaction	Dislikes, resists, overreactive
Motor Skills	Varies, good to poor	Varies, good to poor	Varies, good to poor	Varies, clumsy, poor coordination
Eye Contact	Avoidant	Avoidant-Inconsistent	Avoidant-inconsistent	Poor, inconsistent
Earliest Diagnosis	16–30 months	16–30 months	16–30 months	Preschool
Intelligence	Mental retardation in 75–85 percent	Mental retardation	Varies—may be average	Normal to superior

How common is Asperger's Disorder?

It is difficult to know how many children, teens, and adults have AD. Only recognized in the USA since 1994, there has been limited time for researchers to count the true prevalence.

You may have read about dramatic increases in autism and Autism Spectrum Disorder (ASD). Researchers point to two reasons for this increase. Before AD gained official recognition in 1994, studies counted only autism, finding 4 cases per 10,000. When AD was identified, it was grouped along with autism, and both disorders began to be reported together as the number of individuals with ASD, rather than separate findings for autism and AD. The addition of a third diagnosis, Pervasive Developmental Disorder, Not Otherwise Specified (PDD-NOS), has also been added to the numbers. Children with PDD-NOS have symptoms of autism or Asperger's but not enough to actually be given either diagnosis. They are nonetheless usually counted in the studies and contribute to the rise in the numbers of children reported as having ASD.

The second suspected cause of the dramatic increase in the number of children being diagnosed was the broadening of symptoms that allowed a child to be identified as having autism. Since autism was first included in the *Diagnostic and Statistical Manual of Mental Disorders (DSM)* in 1980 there have been substantial changes in the way the diagnosis is made, allowing more children to meet criteria for diagnosis than in previous years. Many researchers argue that the changes in the diagnostic criteria are responsible for the increases in autism and ASD, refuting the idea that autism and ASD are actually increasing.

These changes in the way diagnoses are made and counted unfortunately make it impossible to know how many individuals truly have AD. We do know that AD is more common than autism, with estimates of AD occurring in 20–25 per 10,000. Rates of autism for many years were reported as 3–4 per 10,000. However, since the recognition of AD, the broadening of autism, and the creation of the term autism spectrum disorders, the numbers have increased dramatically. In 2006 the Center for Disease Control (CDC) reported between 2 and 6 per 1,000 as having ASD. These numbers translate to estimates of 1 per 500 on the low end and 1 per 166 on the high end. This does not mean that 1 in 166 children has autism, as you may have read in many news stories. It is important to understand that the figure of 1 in 166 is the highest estimated number and includes autism, AD, and PDD-NOS. Failure to understand these estimates and the changes in diagnosis gives the false impression that autism is on the rise in epidemic proportions.

While it appears that the estimates of autism may be over-reported, the incidence of AD is probably actually underdiagnosed. Since it is a new disorder, many doctors may not be fully experienced with how to evaluate it. The vague list of symptoms can make it unrecognizable as a disorder, and its overlap with many other disorders may easily cause it to be diagnosed as something else. Until we know more about AD, it will likely remain underdiagnosed.

Is Asperger's Disorder a real disorder?

It is not uncommon for people who do not understand psychological disorders to say that they are not real. You have probably been told everything from "he's just a boy" to "if he were my kid, he would never act that way" to "she is just spoiled." This can be very frustrating and insulting and make you question your perceptions about your child—and maybe even your doctor's diagnosis.

Some argue that AD is not a "disorder" but just an extreme form of normal traits that exist in all of us. Individuals with AD may simply be on the more introverted and socially incapable end of the spectrum. Another theory is that AD is an extreme version of the male brain. Males tend to be more systematic and females more empathic, just the pattern seen in AD.

Others call AD a neurodivergent disorder, meaning those who have it are neurologically different from the average person, whom they call neurotypical. The fact that numerous studies using brain-imaging techniques have found noticeable differences in the brains of individuals with AD when compared to nondisordered individuals argues strongly in favor of AD being a "real" disorder.

Is Asperger's Disorder caused by something in the brain?

There is strong evidence that the cause of AD and ASD lie in the brain. Research studies have repeatedly found differences between the brains of those with AD in comparison to those without. While scientists have yet to locate one particular place in the brain they believe might be responsible, many studies suggest the frontal lobe, which is the area around the forehead. Several studies have also found differences between the brains of children with AD and those with autism. Some studies have shown damage in the right temporal lobe—the area around the temples—of those with AD, and in the left temporal lobe in autistic people. Other studies have found just the opposite pattern, making it difficult to reach conclusions about these findings. Because AD has only been studied in the USA since 1994, there has not been sufficient time to conduct extensive research. Further studies are clearly needed and are underway.

While these studies are promising, it is important to understand that their findings do not mean that brain scanning techniques can diagnose AD. Be cautious about any professional suggesting a brain scan for diagnosing any psychological disorder.

Is Asperger's Disorder genetic?

There is a strong suspicion that AD may be genetic; however, scientists have yet to find a gene. Research shows that AD tends to run in families. If your child has AD, there may be someone else in the family with AD or ASD. Twin studies suggest strong support for a genetic contribution to autism, with greater numbers of autism seen in identical twins when compared to fraternal twins. This pattern is seen both in autism and ASD. When one identical twin has ASD, there is a greater than 90 percent chance that the other twin will have significant features of autism, if not the full disorder.

Scientists are also examining the male chromosome, the Y chromosome. Approximately 80 percent of those with ASD are male, leading researchers to believe problems with the Y chromosome may be a potential cause.

Few adults with autism marry and have children, leaving little opportunity to study the genetics of parent to child. Those with AD, however, commonly marry and bear children. Future research will thus have an opportunity to examine if there is a pattern of AD between parent and child.

What other factors are suspected of causing Asperger's Disorder?

Various causes of AD have been suspected and studied, yet none have been proven. As with diagnosis, AD has been combined with autism in the search for a cause.

Recently, vaccines have been under attack, with parents insisting their child was fine until he was vaccinated and almost immediately afterwards began to shown signs of autism. Research in the USA and various other countries investigated this theory and found no basis to support it. While studies have conclusively determined that the most suspicious agent, thimerosal, is not a cause of autism, the

Federal Drug Administration (FDA) in the USA has nonetheless decreased the amount of this mercury-based preservative in vaccines. Studies looking into other vaccine agents are still being conducted.

Chemicals in the environment are also under investigation as a cause of a variety of childhood disorders, including ASD. To date there is no evidence that chemicals cause AD, ASD, or any childhood disorder.

Maternal factors such as use of prescription medications and conditions during pregnancy are also being investigated. Various medications used in early childhood are also being explored as potential causes. Despite all the research done to date, we still have no concrete answer for what causes AD.

Is there a cure for Asperger's Disorder?

There is no cure for AD. No form of therapy or medication will correct AD. No one outgrows AD or overcomes it. If your child is diagnosed with AD, she will have it for her lifetime. Despite this, however, numerous interventions and treatments can dramatically improve your child's functioning now, and over the long term provide him with tools and skills that will help give him a relatively successful outcome in adulthood.

When thinking of a "cure" for AD, some argue against such a need. A more accepting view of differences in the wide range of human behavior favors a position of embracing AD rather than trying to get rid of it. Even though individuals with AD share similar traits, they are as different as anyone else and have as much to offer the world as any other person. Some would even argue against the words *disorder* and *symptom*, preferring to describe AD in terms of a personality style, traits, and qualities. The thought is that if we try to cure AD, we will miss out on the benefits that individuals with AD have to offer society.

How is Asperger's Disorder treated?

The goal in treatment of AD is to manage the child's symptoms and improve his functioning. Parents seeking a cure or to "change" their child will be disappointed by any form of treatment they obtain. Those who understand that AD is a lifelong disorder and that treatment has its best effects over the long term will be far more satisfied. Improvement in your child happens over the course of years, not weeks or months.

Your child will likely require a variety of treatments during his childhood and adolescence. Treatments shown to be effective in helping children, teens, and families cope with and manage the symptoms of AD include:

- Behavior modification
- Occupational therapy
- Special education
- Social skills therapy
- Speech therapy

Treatment for AD must start early, as soon as the diagnosis is made. It must be intensive, meaning many hours per week and in all environments, including home and school. Training yourself on how to raise a child with AD is critical to the outcome of your child. Parental support is also important as it is very stressful to raise a child with AD. You must be active in your child's treatment, learning the skills and tools your child learns so that you can reinforce them outside of the treatment setting. Treatment must be individualized to meet the specific needs of your child. Generalization of skills learned in treatment is one of the main goals, hence the need for parents to be actively involved. Parents should view themselves as co-therapists, learning all they can from the treatment team so they can be the therapist at home. Applied Behavioral Analysis is a skill parents must learn in order to teach and reinforce appropriate behaviors. AD children should have programs at school to address their symptoms and should be included in the mainstream setting as much as possible.

Can medication help Asperger's Disorder?

There are no medications to treat AD. No medicine is available that will improve the main symptoms of impaired social skills, language, or restricted interests. These symptoms must be addressed with therapy.

Medications are available for several coexisting disorders. Some parents choose medication for their AD child if they also have ADD or ADHD, depression, anxiety, or obsessive-compulsive disorder. There are a variety of medicines for these disorders; however, many are not FDA-approved for children. It is very important that you learn about the medication before giving it to your child. Pharmaceutical companies post information on their websites about the appropriate use of the medication, dosage, ages it is approved for, and side effects.

Sometimes medication is used for a specific symptom even if a child does not have a coexisting disorder. Related behavior problems of aggression, moodiness, inattentiveness, and impulsivity displayed by some AD children can be severe enough that parents opt to use medication. Keep in mind that medication is not a magic pill. It can decrease some of the problematic behaviors, but it is important to understand that medication is one tool, and if used must be done so in conjunction with therapy.

Chapter 2

GETTING YOUR CHILD EVALUATED

- What symptoms signal that my child should be evaluated?
- When it is time to get my child evaluated?
- What should be included in an evaluation?
- Is a diagnosis necessary?
- Should my child have a medical evaluation?
- How do I find a doctor?
- What type of doctor should evaluate my child?
- What should parents know about pediatricians?
- What should parents know about developmental pediatricians?
- What should parents know about child psychiatrists?
- What should parents know about pediatric neurologists?
- What should parents know about clinical psychologists?
- What should parents know about pediatric neuropsychologists?
- What should parents know about educational psychologists?
- What should parents look for in choosing a doctor?
- What tests are used to diagnose Asperger's Disorder?
- Should my child have educational testing?
- Do children behave differently in a one-to-one testing situation?
- What information can an IQ test provide?
- What information can personality testing provide?
- How often should testing be done?
- What information can school achievement tests provide?
- What information can report cards provide?
- Can a diagnosis be made from a behavior checklist?
- Is there a checklist to diagnose Asperger's Disorder?
- What information should I tell the doctor during the evaluation?
- Is family history important in evaluating Asperger's Disorder?
- What records should I give to the doctor?
- What questions will the doctor ask me about my child?
- What if the evaluation is inconclusive?

What symptoms signal that my child should be evaluated?

Parents often suspect that their child is different from other children long before they receive the diagnosis of Asperger's Disorder. Parents of AD children often recall that their child was displaying symptoms as early as preschool. Yet it is hard to come to terms with the idea that your child may have a disorder. It is common to try to minimize and normalize the symptoms your child is displaying. It is also easy to miss the early signs that surface.

Looking back, parents can recall that their AD child showed a noticeable preference for playing alone in preschool. When he did play with other children, he wanted to dominate the play. He was insistent on routine and showed exaggerated upset when changes occurred.

In elementary school, your child may appear to be different, immature, and unusual. An odd gaze, inability to read social cues, poor conversation skills, and obsessive interest in a topic with a tendency to lecture about it are hallmark indicators of AD. Milder forms of AD may not surface until mid or late elementary school, when the inability to fit in with his peers cannot be ignored or explained away.

When is it time to get my child evaluated?

The time to seek an evaluation is as soon as you begin to suspect that your child does not function or behave like other children his age. Observations from teachers, relatives, friends, and other parents may be your first indication that your child may have AD. Repeated feedback from others, even if you don't agree, should warrant an evaluation. Even if a diagnosis is not determined at the time, symptoms can be defined and interventions can begin. Research repeatedly shows that the earlier the detection and treatment, the better the long-term outcome for the child and family.

Unfortunately, many parents are reluctant to seek an evaluation and hold out hope that their child will outgrow the symptoms, believing it to be a phase. The average age a child is diagnosed with AD is ten to eleven years. What makes this so alarming is that the average parent began to suspect problems when their child was two and a half years old, resulting in their child going eight or nine years without services. Research suggests that 10 percent of individuals with AD are not diagnosed until after the age of twenty, going their entire childhood without services.

What should be included in an evaluation?

Evaluation for AD is not as simple as other childhood disorders. Because AD affects so many areas of your child's life, a team approach to diagnosis is best. Your child should be evaluated in each of the areas that AD impacts. Each specialist is an expert in their area, and no one professional can assess all areas of your child's functioning. Early and thorough assessment will ensure that your child has a comprehensive treatment plan that will address every area where he has weaknesses. It is tempting to stop having your child evaluated once he is diagnosed; however, diagnosis is only the beginning. Diagnosis in itself tells only a small part of the story of your child's functioning. Knowing he has AD is the first step in getting you on the road to obtaining the appropriate types of evaluation that will determine where he is functioning in impacted areas and what types of intervention he needs. Early and thorough evaluation also provides a baseline from which you can judge progress throughout his childhood and adolescence.

A thorough evaluation should include all of the following:

- Medical examination
- Psychological evaluation
- Intellectual assessment
- Speech and language assessment
- Learning disorders evaluation
- Neurological examination
- Neuropsychological testing

Is a diagnosis necessary?

A diagnosis describes a group of symptoms and provides a concise vocabulary for educators, parents, physicians, and mental health professionals to use. Of course, a diagnosis does not tell all there is to know about a child, yet knowing your child has formally been diagnosed with AD provides a tremendous amount of information and helps explain his behavior. Once you learn about AD, you can respond to your child in helpful ways. You can also become aware of problems caused by AD that you might otherwise fail to recognize, dismiss as just a phase, or misinterpret as willful disobedience or social rudeness. The earlier a diagnosis is made the sooner you can take advantage of early intervention programs that are specifically designed for AD.

A formal diagnosis is not always necessary. If symptoms can be identified and interventions planned, a diagnosis may not have to be made. However, there are situations when a diagnosis is required. When seeking reimbursement from insurance, a diagnosis is always required. Special education services require the presence of a disorder that impairs learning. Some children have symptoms of AD that are not severe enough to be diagnosed as AD, yet they can nonetheless benefit from an evaluation and treatment.

Should my child have a medical evaluation?

There are no medical tests to determine if a child or teen has AD. Unlike a medical condition where a blood, X-ray, or CT scan test provides exact answers, AD has no definitive test. Despite some physicians using such medical techniques as EEG or QEEG (Electroencephalogram and Quantitative Electroencephalogram), no medical test currently exists that can determine if someone has AD. Such procedures are not supported by the vast majority of physicians for the purpose of diagnosing AD.

All children should see a pediatrician for regular checkups and vaccinations. Children with AD tend to have more unusual medical conditions than the average child and thus need a thorough medical evaluation. Some children with AD will need to be referred by their pediatrician to a medical specialist depending on their particular medical condition. Estimates of 12–37 percent of children with AD may have one of the following medical disorders:

- Chromosomal abnormalities
- Thyroid disorder
- Neurological disorders
- Neurofibromatosis (soft tumors all over the body)
- Tuberous sclerosis (tumorlike growths on the brain, retina, or viscera)

How do I find a doctor?

Finding an experienced physician or mental health professional with expertise in evaluating AD is one of the most important decisions you will make as a parent. Some parents shy away from professionals who specialize in AD, believing the expert will see the disorder in every child. This fear results in evaluations performed by less experienced professionals unfamiliar with AD. Experts in AD do not diagnose AD simply because that is their expertise. They have seen numerous children with AD and have seen the infinite number of ways the symptoms manifest. An expert professional provides the best opportunity to obtain an accurate evaluation.

Referrals from others are the best way to find an expert. Seek out agencies and professionals that have special knowledge about AD. Ask people you know for a recommendation. Your child's teacher, principal, and pediatrician are likely good sources for recommendations. Parents with children already diagnosed with AD are usually excellent resources for referrals. Awareness of AD is growing, and the Internet provides easy access to information and can be a good source to find local and national AD organizations which may lead you to specialists. You will find some of these listed in the Appendix.

What type of doctor should evaluate my child?

There are a variety of professionals who are qualified to evaluate children for AD. The most important thing about who you choose is not so much what their degree is, but rather that they have ample experience evaluating children for AD.

Professionals who evaluate for AD are:

- Pediatricians
- Developmental Pediatricians
- Psychiatrists
- Pediatric Neurologists
- Clinical Psychologists
- Pediatric Neuropsychologists
- Educational Psychologists

While every professional will use the criteria listed in the *Diagnostic and Statistical Manual of Mental Disorders Fourth Edition-*

Text Revision (DSM-IV-TR), each will have his own tools and procedures and threshold for what level of symptoms he thinks meets criteria for the diagnosis.

When selecting which type of evaluator will asses your child, there will be pros and cons for each. Pediatricians tend to have limited time. However, your pediatrician likely knows your child quite well and has a long-standing history of observing her. Psychiatrists, neurologists, and developmental pediatricians will all likely perform a longer evaluation, but they can only offer medication treatment. Pediatric neuropsychologists and educational psychologists provide testing but typically do not offer treatment. Clinical psychologists, many of whom can provide testing if necessary, can evaluate and provide treatment.

What should parents know about pediatricians?

Pediatricians are medical doctors who have an MD and have completed four years of medical school in addition to an internship and residency in their area of specialty. Pediatricians evaluate, diagnose, and treat childhood medical illnesses, as well as monitor the development of children as they grow.

Parents often turn to their pediatrician when they notice their child is having behavioral difficulties or does not seem to be keeping up with his age-mates in developing skills. The advantage of seeing a pediatrician is that they see hundreds of children and know what behavior is typical and what behavior is outside the norm. They know at what age children should be developing various skills. While some pediatricians are skilled in evaluating AD, most of them structure their practice for short visits with an eye toward quick evaluation and treatment. Pediatric practices are usually not designed for the lengthy interviews necessary to evaluate AD; however, they are a good source for a referral for a more in-depth evaluation by another specialist. Do not be surprised if your pediatrician is not very experienced with AD. Being a relatively newly recognized disorder, some pediatricians may not have yet gained the expertise in AD.

What should parents know about developmental pediatricians?

A developmental pediatrician is a medical doctor with a specialty in evaluating abnormalities in development and behavior in infants, toddlers, and children. These pediatricians are specialists in assessing a child's cognitive, social, behavioral, and physical development. Unlike a general pediatrician who primarily treats medical conditions in children, these specialists focus on the abnormal medical, psychological, neurological, genetic, behavioral, social, and developmental disorders of childhood.

Developmental pediatricians perform a physical examination, looking for medical causes of problems. They evaluate physical growth, motor development, and nutritional needs. They are skilled in screening for cognitive and speech and language delays. They also assess social and emotional development along with adaptive development. A typical initial evaluation with a developmental pediatrician is comprehensive and lengthy, and it is not uncommon for the appointment to last two hours or more. Because they are experts in the complete development of children, they take a team approach to the child and will typically advise parents to seek additional evaluation and treatment with various other professionals. They can usually provide referrals to such specialists and can coordinate with each professional, serving as a case manager who keeps an eye on the overall treatment plan for your child.

What should parents know about child psychiatrists?

A child psychiatrist is a medical doctor who specializes in the evaluation and treatment of childhood and adolescent behavioral and psychological disorders. Psychiatrists generally allow for at least one-hour interviews in their evaluation, with an eye toward the diagnosis and determination of medication needs. The majority of psychiatrists prescribe medication as their sole form of treatment and do not provide psychotherapy or behavioral treatment. Many psychiatrists, however, will educate parents regarding the need for psychological and behavioral treatment. After the initial evaluation, the psychiatrist will schedule follow-up appointments to assess the effectiveness and the side effects of the medication. Once the medication is stable, most psychiatrists will have follow-up appointments every three to six months.

Because there is no medication to treat AD, your child may never require the services of a psychiatrist. Some children and teens with AD have a secondary diagnosis that is responsive to medication, such as ADHD or depression. In such cases, a psychiatrist may be appropriate if you are considering medication as an addition to your child's treatment plan. Some children with AD do not have a second disorder but have behavior problems that may be severe enough to warrant a psychiatric evaluation.

What should parents know about pediatric neurologists?

A pediatric neurologist is a medical doctor who diagnoses and treats disorders of the nervous system in children and adolescents. This includes diseases of the brain, spinal cord, nerves, and muscles. A pediatric neurologist may serve as a consultant to other physicians as well as provide long-term care to patients with chronic neurological disorders. Any child diagnosed with AD or thought to have AD should see a pediatric neurologist to evaluate their neurological functioning. Neurologists perform tests of nerve functioning by having the child engage in specific motor and mental tasks. If brain or central nervous system dysfunction is suspected, the neurologist may suggest an EEG, CT, MRI, or other scans of the brain. These tests are not necessary in an evaluation for AD and cannot determine the presence or absence of AD, but they may be necessary to evaluate other nervous system disorders, which tend to be more frequent in children with AD than nondisordered children. If a condition is present, the neurologist will provide medical treatment and monitoring. Once your child is given a clean bill of nervous system health, he generally will not see the neurologist again. Neurologists will likely be able to provide you with a referral for psychological and behavioral treatment.

What should parents know about clinical psychologists?

Clinical psychologists have a PhD or PsyD, typically in clinical or counseling psychology. They provide evaluation, testing, and treatment. Evaluation by a clinical psychologist will focus on determining the cause of the symptoms displayed. At least one hour is scheduled for the evaluation. This includes a history, a review of the child's report cards and academic achievement tests, observation of the child, behavioral analysis, and an interview of the parents and child.

The clinical psychologist may or may not administer tests to your child as part of the diagnostic procedure. Testing, although it provides useful information, does not definitively tell if your child has AD. Instead, the test results will be used by the psychologist as just one piece of her evaluation.

Treatment provided by clinical psychologists includes various forms of psychotherapy. This includes individual, group, family, and couples treatment. Clinical psychologists who specialize in AD are generally specialists in behavior modification and thus can provide parent education and training. They are also likely to provide social skills training for your child. Psychologists may offer all the necessary forms of treatment in their practice or be able to provide referrals to the other types of specialists.

What should parents know about pediatric neuropsychologists?

A pediatric neuropsychologist has a PhD, usually in clinical or counseling psychology with postdoctoral specialty training in neuropsychology. These specialists study the individual functions of the brain and are able to evaluate a child's abilities in highly specific skills. For example, they not only evaluate a child's memory functioning but can also assess their memory for visual, auditory, immediate, and short- and long-term abilities. Testing includes paper and pencil tests, oral tests, and tests requiring the manipulation of objects.

Neuropsychological testing is not done for purposes of diagnosing AD but to provide in-depth evaluation of your child's cognitive functioning. Motor, memory, organization, planning, problem-solving, and visual-perceptual skills are among the many brain functions a neuropsychologist tests. Not only are the test scores useful in measuring strengths and weaknesses, but how your child approaches each task will be carefully watched to make observations on your child's preferred style of learning as well as the unique way in which he solves various mental tasks. Results will be prepared in a report with recommendations in the form of interventions to be carried out in the classroom and during homework. Teachers, tutors, and educational therapists can then create lessons geared towards your child's specific cognitive functioning.

What should parents know about educational psychologists?

Educational psychologists have a master's or doctorate degree in education, an MEd or EdD. They may evaluate and diagnose AD, but more often they focus on the evaluation and treatment of learning disorders and learning problems.

Educational psychologists perform evaluations through a variety of educational tests, including IQ and academic achievement tests. They are skilled at making very specific recommendations based upon those test results. Recommendations are designed for classroom and homework time. Educational psychologists are experts at applying those recommendations in a one-on-one setting with the student through educational therapy. They can also provide assistance in the design of a special education program.

Educational therapy is a process that combines an understanding of how learning takes place in the brain with the knowledge of specialized teaching methods that help children learn. Educational psychologists can help children with AD who do not have a learning disorder but still have difficulties with homework, organization and planning of projects, or studying.

Due to budget and time constraints, the educational psychologist employed by your child's school will not provide the comprehensive testing and recommendations that a private-practice educational psychologist can. Nor can they provide the educational therapy that a private practitioner can.

What should parents look for in choosing a doctor?

Not only is it difficult to choose which *type* of doctor to evaluate your child, it is equally as difficult to choose *who* that doctor will be. One of the most important factors in selecting your child's doctor is to find out whether or not he or she is able to view your child's entire functioning and develop a comprehensive treatment plan. Will the doctor take the time to review your child's records? Can the doctor provide referrals to address each of your child's needs? Will he work cooperatively with the other members of your child's treatment team, including the teacher?

It may not be easy to find a doctor who is experienced with AD. One of the best ways to choose a doctor is through a recommendation from others who know of the doctor's work and reputation. View their website and read their brochures in order to learn about their degree, area of practice, specialties, philosophy of treatment, and interventions they are able to provide. Once you have found a doctor that you think might be right for your child, you are ready to schedule an appointment asking for an evaluation to determine if your child has AD.

What tests are used to diagnose AD?

When parents are advised that they should have their child "tested" for AD what they really are being told is they should have their child evaluated. Testing refers to specific laboratory exams that give exact answers to whether or not something exists, such as a bladder infection or a broken bone. No medical test currently exits that can determine if someone has AD. There are some medical tests, however, that your child's pediatrician or neurologist may recommend in order to rule out physical causes of your child's symptoms.

There are also no psychological or educational tests that will definitively determine if a child has AD. However, there are several checklists and tests specifically designed to aid in the evaluation of AD. You and your child's teacher may be asked to complete one or more questionnaires as part of the evaluation process. In addition to a detailed history, observation of your child, a review of his records, and a behavioral analysis, psychological and educational testing can be helpful as part of the diagnostic evaluation.

Should my child have educational testing?

The most common reason to use educational testing in an evaluation for AD is to determine if a learning disorder is present. AD children often have very scattered academic abilities that cause them to appear brilliant in some areas and surprisingly incapable in others. Without the type of information that educational testing provides, it can be quite difficult for your child's teacher to set appropriate expectations for your child.

To determine if a learning disorder or weakness is present, the evaluator will administer a standardized IQ test; the most commonly used being the Wechsler tests, of which there are preschool, elementary/middle school, and high school/adult versions. These tests are not the same as paper-and-pencil IQ tests sold at bookstores and on the Internet; these are the gold standard for accurate IQ testing and occur face-to-face.

A learning disorder evaluation will also include an academic achievement test battery. These are also administered face-to-face, directly to the child by the psychologist. Commonly used tests include Woodcock Johnson III, Kaufman, and Peabody Individual Achievement Test. If your child's IQ is significantly higher than his academic achievement, he may be considered to have a learning disorder.

Do children behave differently in a one-to-one testing situation?

When testing is introduced into the diagnostic evaluation, you may be concerned that the results are distorted because of the one-to-one interaction. Typically, children do better in a one-to-one situation when compared to the classroom or during homework. This is actually an asset to the diagnostic evaluation. The benefit provided by one-to-one testing is the psychologist's ability to measure the child's true abilities. Without the distractions of the classroom, and with the added novelty of meeting with the psychologist, children generally enjoy the testing and try hard to please the evaluator. This allows the psychologist to measure what the child truly knows, even if his knowledge is not reflected in his work or on his report cards.

The second benefit of one-to-one testing is that because it takes four to eight hours to complete, the psychologist is usually able to observe the child in several different sessions. Once the novelty wears off and the desire to please becomes hard to sustain, the child eventually displays his typical behavior. Even under the ideal situation of a quiet office and one-to-one attention, children with AD can't help but display their symptoms.

What information can an IQ test provide?

Children with AD appear to be far smarter than their classmates. Their superb vocabulary and excellent long-term memory for facts often impress adults. Advanced intellect might be thought of only as an asset; however, their superior intelligence often is used against them. Adults cannot imagine why on Earth the AD child behaves the way he does when he is so smart. "You should know better!" is a frequent scolding for the AD child—who actually does not know better! Just because he has the vocabulary of a college graduate does not mean he can refrain from announcing to the class that he finds the teacher boring.

IQ testing will give you and your child's teacher a picture of how intellectually *capable* your child is in a wide variety of areas, including long-term learning, immediate memory, social judgment, understanding cause and effect, and abstract thinking, among others. It is not uncommon to find that despite impressive verbal skills, the AD child has an average IQ. Generally, he will have areas where he is superior, some where he is average, and others below average.

Knowing his strengths and weaknesses can eliminate the pressure for him to perform well on everything.

What information can personality testing provide?

Psychological testing, or personality testing as it is sometimes called, provides a wealth of information about a child's psychological functioning. While no psychological test can determine if your child has AD, it can assist in the evaluation. A battery of tests will give the psychologist a look inside your child's emotional world. Aspects of your child's personality that would take months to observe can be picked up in a few hours of psychological testing. His social style, coping skills, world outlook, problem-solving style, mood, and self-esteem can be determined by psychological test results. The subtle forms of anxiety and depression that AD children often have are not easily observed, yet can readily be discovered during psychological testing.

This type of testing involves activities that most children find enjoyable, such as drawing pictures, telling stories about pictures, and completing sentences. As children get older, they are able to take self-report tests where they can answer questions about their thoughts, feelings, and behavior. Psychological testing should include several tests to obtain a comprehensive picture. Results can be immensely helpful for the psychotherapist working with your child in providing an in-depth picture of your child's internal world. Interventions can be designed specifically for your child based upon the test results.

How often should testing be done?

Unlike certain medical tests that have a standard time frame to repeat, there is no set schedule of when IQ, academic achievement, neuropsychological, or psychological testing should be done. Once a test battery is completed, the benefit of readministering the tests at a later date is to measure progress. Most psychologists would say that at least one year should pass before testing is repeated. This may even be too soon as progress with learning disorders and AD is slow, and measurable success may not show up after one year. Two to three years is a more reasonable time frame that allows the child to benefit from the academic, behavioral, and psychological interventions. There can be exceptions to this general recommendation. If testing is to be done more frequently, there should be a specific purpose and a plan for modifying interventions based upon the results. Retesting should involve a comparison of both sets of test data. Having the same psychologist administer the retesting has the advantage of his experience with and prior knowledge of the child. If you choose a different psychologist for a retest, be sure they are provided with the previous test data and written report so they may do an accurate comparison.

What information can school achievement tests provide?

Each year, schools administer standardized academic achievement tests in a paper-and-pencil format that an entire class takes at the same time. The most common tests are the STAR, SAT, CAT-9, and CTBS. These tests provide a measure of what the child has learned in school in the past year in various academic areas. They are not a substitute for the individually administered academic achievement tests, but are a useful measure of how the child is progressing from year to year in the basic subject areas.

It is important to bring all of your child's annual academic achievement test scores to an evaluator. This will help determine if testing for a learning disorder is necessary. It will also help in recommendations for academic placement. It is not unusual to have a child with AD be near failing in school but have annual achievement test scores in the ninetieth percentile. His report card reflects homework and what he does in class, while the academic achievement tests measure what he actually learned. Comparing his scores with his report card can help determine if his problems lie more in learning or in behavior.

What information can report cards provide?

Report cards are often mistaken for a measure of the child's learning throughout the school year. However, these are more a measure of a child's performance, and only partially reflect his learning. Instead, academic achievement tests tell what a child has *learned*. Report cards largely tell how the child did in producing and completing work, being accurate in his answers, writing properly, and cooperating with the teacher, among other skills.

It is not unusual for some children with AD to have poor report cards. Despite their average to above average intelligence and lack of learning disorders, the challenges of the classroom can be too much for some children, and this is reflected in their poor performance. Their grades may vary widely from A's in some subjects to F's in others.

Other AD children may perform well academically but have grave difficulties with citizenship, cooperation, work habits, and classroom functioning. Of particular interest on report cards are the teacher comments. Notes written by teachers on report cards provide valuable information to your child's doctor. Their comments can shed light on how the symptoms of AD are displayed in the classroom and can be helpful in diagnosis and in treatment planning.

Can a diagnosis be made from a behavior checklist?

Checklists are standardized questionnaires that list a wide variety of behaviors that children engage in. Many parents are alarmed when their doctor relies on a behavior checklist in diagnosing AD. While this should not be the sole source of information, the checklists can be a very useful diagnostic tool. While it is quick for parents to fill out and quick for doctors to score and interpret, years of research have gone on behind the scenes to develop these checklists and make them useful.

Here's how they work. Researchers provide a lengthy list of behaviors that children engage in. They find very large groups of parents to complete the questionnaires. By having thousands of parents who have children free of problems complete the questionnaires, the researchers are able to see what so-called normal children look like in terms of mood and behavior. By having thousands of parents whose children have disorders complete the checklists, they are able to see how children with a variety of problems appear on the checklist. Your child's test scores are examined to see if he more closely matches the "normal" group or the Asperger's group. Your child's scores will also be compared to other disordered groups such as the depressed, anxious, hyperactive, inattentive, aggressive, and socially problematic groups.

Is there a checklist to diagnose Asperger's Disorder?

There are no checklists that can say for certain if a child has AD. However, in recent years there have been questionnaires developed that are good at screening which children *might* have AD. Parents, teachers, and others who know the child fill out a short written questionnaire about the child's social, emotional, communication, cognitive, motor skills, and interest patterns. Children who score high on these screening instruments should have a more thorough evaluation to determine if they have AD and/or another disorder.

Some of the commonly used screening tests include:

- Australian Scale for Asperger's Syndrome
- Autism Spectrum Disorders Screening Questionnaire
- Asperger's Syndrome Diagnostic Scale
- Gilliam's Asperger's Disorder Scale
- Childhood Asperger's Syndrome Test
- Autism-Spectrum Quotient

If your doctor uses checklists, they should include additional questionnaires that ask about a wide variety of behaviors, not just AD. Even if you are reasonably sure that your child has AD, it is very important that he is evaluated for other disorders. Some of the checklists that are commonly used to evaluate children for a wide variety of behavioral and psychological disorders include:

- Achenbach Child Behavior Checklist
- Conner's Rating Scale
- Achenbach Teacher Report Form

What information should I tell the doctor during the evaluation?

Preparing for an evaluation or meeting with a new doctor is very important. Pediatricians are especially limited on their time, with the average office visit lasting only ten minutes. Psychologists and psychiatrists typically have an average visit of one hour. There is a lot of information to cover in ten to sixty minutes. Organization and preparation can help ensure a thorough evaluation. Use your child's baby book to get specific ages your child achieved various skills.

Prepare to tell the evaluator about your child's:

- Prenatal history
- Early social behavior
- Early language and communication skills
- Early motor skills
- Medical history
- Mental health history
- Medication history
- Behavior history
- Academic history

Many evaluators have lengthy questionnaires for parents to fill out prior to the visit. While this exhausts some parents, it can save time and allows the doctor to focus her interview on the most relevant questions. Try to be brief but specific in what you observe in your child. Bring a list of symptoms and problems you observe in your child and be prepared to provide a few examples of how, when, and where each symptom occurs.

Is family history important in evaluating AD?

Because many disorders run in families, your evaluator will take a family history. Family history is equally important in diagnosing a disorder as it is in ruling it out. It is important that your child's evaluator know about your family history to determine if there are other causes or contributors to your child's symptoms. Knowing where your child came from genetically and environmentally is part of who he is and cannot be separated out from his symptoms. You do not have to disclose names of family members, but it is helpful for the evaluator to know about the history of both the child's mother's and father's families. Prepare ahead of time and gather the necessary information to answer questions about your child's family history. Background about siblings, parents, grandparents, and aunts and uncles can be useful in the following categories:

- Mental health history
- History of AD
- Substance abuse history
- Criminal history
- School and learning history
- Behavior problems
- Mood and/or behavior medication history
- Suicide history
- Highest grade completed
- Divorce and stepfamily constellation
- Trauma history

What records should I give to the doctor?

Your child's records are an essential piece of the information needed to perform a diagnostic evaluation. AD in particular is a disorder that relies heavily on a thorough history taking. Without records, the evaluator can rely only on what you tell him and what he observes in his office.

The following records are important for your doctor to consider in the diagnostic evaluation:

- Report cards
- Annual academic achievement test scores
- Individual education plans
- Notes sent home from school
- Educational testing reports
- Personality testing reports
- AD prior evaluation results

The easier you make it for your doctor to review the records the more likely it is that they will take the time to read them. Prepare a copy of all the records for the doctor to keep in her file. Call the doctor's office and ask if you may send the records prior to the evaluation in case the doctor has time to review them before your visit. Organize your records by category and place them in order from oldest to most recent. This way the doctor can see the changes in your child from year to year by simply turning to the next page.

What questions will the doctor ask me about my child?

Much of the information your doctor needs will be contained in the records you send or bring with you, the behavior checklist you complete, and the history questionnaire you fill out. Combined, these help your doctor narrow down the questions he will ask you. You can assist your doctor by being an accurate and concise reporter. Bring a list of the behaviors you observe in your child and be sure to tell the doctor about them.

Be prepared to provide information regarding how well your child is able to:

- Play with age-mates
- Make eye contact
- Have a conversation
- Handle changes
- Use imaginative play
- Understand what others are thinking and feeling
- Use language without errors
- Use facial expressions to communicate feelings
- Display interest in a wide variety of topics and objects
- Understand and respond to social cues
- Show interest in others
- Speak in a normal voice
- Cope with noise
- Make and keep friends
- Manage his anger
- Display a sense of humor
- Understand body language
- Understand unspoken rules of socializing
- Generalize lessons from one situation
- Recognize when he hurts someone's feelings
- Understand figures of speech
- Show emotional maturity
- Be aware of how his behavior impacts others
- Manage her feelings

What if the evaluation is inconclusive?

It is not uncommon to have a diagnostic evaluation be inconclusive. Because AD is based on clinical judgment, there are cases where one doctor will determine AD is present but another doctor will say it is not. Your child may be too young to determine if AD is fully present, or the symptoms may not be severe enough to warrant the diagnosis. Doctors differ on where they draw the line for diagnosing. This is not surprising and merely highlights the subjective nature of diagnosing this disorder. In fact, AD is one of the more commonly misdiagnosed disorders because its symptoms are not clear-cut and overlap with both normal behaviors and those of other disorders.

If your child's evaluation is inconclusive, you may opt to obtain a second opinion with the same type of doctor who performed the first evaluation, thus having two opinions from two different psychologists. Alternatively, you may seek a different category of specialist, thus having an opinion, for example, from one psychologist and one psychiatrist. Or as many parents do, you can simply choose to have your child treated for the various problems he exhibits and wait to see if the diagnosis becomes clearer over time.

Chapter 3

COEXISTING DISORDERS

- Is it really Asperger's Disorder or is it something else?
- How do I tell if my child has a second disorder?
- What is ADD?
- What is ADHD?
- What is Obsessive-Compulsive Disorder?
- What is Anxiety Disorder?
- What is Oppositional Defiant Disorder?
- What is Childhood Depression?
- What is Pervasive Developmental Disorder?
- What is Mental Retardation?
- What is Schizoid Personality Disorder?
- What is Reactive Attachment Disorder?
- What is Sensory Integration Disorder?
- What is Developmental Coordination Disorder?
- What is a Communication Disorder?
- What is a learning disorder?
- What is Social Phobia?
- What is Tourette's Disorder?
- What are Enuresis and Encopresis?
- What is a nonverbal learning disorder?
- What is Semantic Pragmatic Disorder?
- What is Gifted and Twice Exceptional?

Is it really Asperger's Disorder or is it something else?

AD is a relatively new disorder, first being included in the mental health professionals' diagnostic book, the 1994 version of *Diagnostic and Statistical Manual-IV-TR*, or *DSM IV-TR* for short. Because it is a new disorder, AD is usually not on the top of the list of disorders that most doctors consider. This can be helpful in that children are not likely to be misdiagnosed with AD when they actually have a different disorder. However, it simultaneously results in children who truly have AD being diagnosed with a different disorder. Because the symptoms of AD are vague, other conditions can easily be mistaken for this disorder. It is therefore very important that a child who appears to have AD be evaluated for other disorders as well.

The most difficult disorder to distinguish from AD is high-functioning autism, as discussed in chapter 1. In addition to other disorders, your doctor must distinguish between whether your child is going through a phase or is having a reaction to a dramatic change in life, such as divorce, trauma, or abuse. Finally, it is more common than not for children with AD to have at least one other disorder. Oftentimes, the second disorder overshadows the symptoms of AD so much so that AD might be missed altogether.

How do I tell if my child has a second disorder?

Most children with AD have additional problems beyond AD. Many have a second disorder, or at a minimum they have additional symptoms that are significant enough that they will require evaluation and treatment from multiple specialists. Because AD has symptoms in the areas of emotions, socialization, thinking, behavior, and communication, a team approach to evaluating your child is essential. Typically, one category of symptoms stands out above the rest, prompting parents to seek evaluation from a specialist, but once diagnosed, they look no further. It is hard enough to accept that your child has one disorder, let alone considering that the problem you just got diagnosed is really just one indication of a more serious disorder or just one of several disorders your child has. It is also daunting to think of the cost of evaluations and testing by multiple specialists. Yet without overcoming the emotional and financial obstacles to a thorough assessment of your child, you are beginning a journey with only a partial road map. Both parents and professionals must be aware that most psychological disorders in children rarely exist in isolation. Without an intellectual, psychological, language, social, and behavioral assessment, not only can other symptoms be overlooked, but additional disorders can be missed.

What is ADD?

Attention Deficit Hyperactivity Disorder-Inattentive Type is more commonly called ADD. It is a disruptive behavior disorder whose symptoms include:

- Inattention
- Distractibility
- Forgetfulness
- Trouble sustaining mental effort
- Repeated mistakes
- Frequent loss of belongings
- Daydreaming or spaciness

Symptoms of ADD may start as early as kindergarten, where the child has trouble playing quietly, sharing toys, taking his nap, and listening. As the ADD child moves into the second, third, and fourth grade, the symptoms become more apparent, with their greatest impact seen in the classroom and during homework. Incomplete work, lying about having homework, tantrums, procrastinating, sloppy work, and losing the necessary homework items are almost daily occurrences.

Although the exact numbers are not known, it is quite common to see ADD coexist with AD. It is also not unusual for the two disorders to be mistaken for one another. The inattentiveness, day-dreaming, and high distractibility of ADD can mimic the lack of interest and empathy for others seen in AD. Additionally, because most children with ADD have poor social skills, as a matter of course AD is not often considered as a coexisting disorder. If your child is diagnosed with ADD, it is important that the doctor also assess for AD.

What is ADHD?

Attention Deficit Hyperactivity Disorder-Hyperactive-Impulsive Type is typically referred to as ADHD. It is a disruptive behavior disorder characterized by:

- Excessive physical activity
- Impulsivity
- Restlessness, fidgeting
- Intrusiveness
- Excessive talking

These children are excessive in their behaviors. They move too much, talk too much, interrupt others, intrude on others' games, cannot settle down, and seem to be driven by an endless motor. Typically they have these symptoms in addition to those of ADD. These symptoms result in a child who is frequently breaking the rules at home, at school, and on the playground, and consequently is not favored by adults or peers.

Symptoms of ADHD often appear in the toddler years, with the first sign most often being the child's constant and seemingly endless physical motion. His inability to take turns in play and conversation looks very much like the lack of empathy seen in AD.

Symptoms of ADHD are quite often seen in children with AD, and many are diagnosed with both disorders. Estimates are so wide in range that they are useless, with various studies reporting ranges from 17 percent to 85 percent of children with AD also having ADHD. Because the symptoms of ADHD are so obvious and difficult to live with, they often overshadow those of AD. AD often goes undetected in ADHD children because both the parents and the evaluator fail to consider it. Any child with ADHD who has problems with social skills should also be evaluated for AD.

What is Obsessive-Compulsive Disorder?

Obsessive-Compulsive Disorder (OCD) is marked by recurrent obsessions and compulsions that interfere with daily functioning. Obsessions are recurrent and persistent ideas, thoughts, impulses, or images that are intrusive and cause distress. The thoughts are unwanted and not within the child or teen's control and go excessively beyond normal worries. Compulsions are repetitive behaviors which serve the sole purpose of preventing or reducing anxiety. The child or teen feels driven to perform the behavior, sometimes to prevent a dreaded result, such as washing hands in order to prevent disease. Some obsessions include performing rigid or stereotyped behaviors that have no real function or connection to preventing the dreaded event.

Because both OCD and AD involve single-minded pursuits and unusual interests, it can be difficult to tell the two disorders apart. While the symptoms of intense preoccupation with a thought or interest can look identical in the two disorders, there are easily identifiable differences. Individuals with OCD do not have the notice-able social difficulties that are a primary problem for those with AD. Nor do they have problems with language. Lastly, the repetitive ideas and behaviors experienced by the AD child are pleasurable and purposely pursued, whereas the OCD child experiences them as unwanted and distressing and tries to resist engaging in them.

What is Anxiety Disorder?

Generalized Anxiety Disorder in children and teens is characterized by persistent and excessive worry that lasts for at least six months. Symptoms of anxiety include:

- Excessive worry
- Difficulty controlling the worry
- Feeling restless or on edge
- Easily fatigued
- Difficulty concentrating
- Irritability
- Muscle tension
- Sleep disturbance

All children have worries from time to time, but children with Generalized Anxiety Disorder are excessively worried and the symptoms are significantly distressing and cause impairment in functioning. The most common worries for children are school or sports performance, and catastrophic events such as earthquakes. Anxious children tend to be perfectionists and may need excessive reassurance.

AD and anxiety disorders are not easily mistaken for one another. However, a child with AD may have an anxiety disorder that is over-looked. Although we do not know how many children with AD have an anxiety disorder, research studies do show that they have more anxiety disorders than children with other types of psychological conditions and more anxiety than the general population of children. These findings are true as young as preschool and become more prevalent as AD children grow.

What is Oppositional Defiant Disorder?

Oppositional Defiant Disorder (ODD) is a recurrent pattern of defiant, disobedient, oppositional, negative, and hostile behavior towards adults. Children with ODD have four or more of the following symptoms:

- Spiteful or vindictive
- Loses temper
- Angry and resentful
- Argues with adults
- Touchy or easily annoyed
- Actively defies or refuses to comply with adults' requests or rules
- Blames others for her mistakes or misbehavior
- Deliberately annoys people

Symptoms must be present for at least six months and occur more frequently than is typical for age and developmental level. The ODD child is a very difficult child to raise; refusing to comply with even the most basic request. She wants her way and there are few things that will stop her from getting it. They live by the philosophy of "you're not the boss of me!" Constant battles result in a cycle of negativity between the parent and the child, and they tend to bring out the worst in one another. The rigidity, insistence on routine, and lack of empathy seen in AD can either mimic ODD or be severe enough that the child is also diagnosed with ODD.

What is Childhood Depression?

Children are usually unaware of what depression is and are unlikely to verbalize it very well. Instead they show their depression in complaints of not feeling well, irritable moods, and social withdrawal. Teens are more aware of their mood and therefore may be more vocal about their depression. Symptoms of depression include:

- Depressed or irritable mood
- Decreased interest or pleasure in activities
- Changes in weight or appetite
- Insomnia or excessive sleeping
- Physical agitation or retardation
- Fatigue or loss of energy
- Feelings of worthlessness or guilt
- Decreased concentration
- Thoughts of death or suicide

Rather than an abrupt change from a usually happy mood to a sad mood, children with AD have a more subtle and slowly emerging onset of depression. Their sadness stems from a daily life of not fitting in, being teased and rejected by their peers, annoying their classmates, and upsetting their parents. As the child grows from year to year, he becomes more aware of his differences from others and his inability to fit in, leading to increased risk for depression as he moves through childhood to adolescence. Suicidal thoughts are not uncommon and must be treated seriously and not regarded as an attempt for attention.

What is Pervasive Developmental Disorder?

Pervasive Developmental Disorder (PDD) is a group of disorders that are characterized by severe impairment in several areas of development. AD is one of the five types of PDD, all of which include significant problems in:

- Reciprocal social interaction
- Communication and language
- Stereotyped behaviors, interests, and activities

In addition to AD, the other PDD include Autistic Disorder, Rett's Disorder, Childhood Disintegrative Disorder, and PDD Not Otherwise Specified. If your child's diagnostic symptoms are not clear, she may be diagnosed with PDD Not Otherwise Specified, which is a label for children who clearly have developmental problems but do not fall into the other PDD classifications.

Autistic Disorder, described in chapter 1, is the most difficult disorder to distinguish from AD. Rett's Disorder is seen only in females and appears after normal development in the first five months of life. There is a measurable slowing in the growth of the head as well as loss of motor skills. AD is more common in males than females and shows no delays in head growth.

Childhood Disintegrative Disorder appears after two years of normal development followed by noticeable loss of skills in language, socialization, movement, self-help, or toileting. AD children do not show a loss of such skills or disturbances in their abilities.

What is Mental Retardation?

Mental Retardation (MR) is diagnosed in individuals with an IQ below 70 who also have significant limitations in self-help skills. Causes of MR are numerous and can often be traced to genetics; prenatal conditions such as toxicity, infections, and trauma; birth complications; and postnatal medical conditions.

Problems in self-help skills are noticed far earlier than IQ deficits. Self-help skills are often referred to as adaptive functioning or adaptive living skills. You may encounter these terms in your child's evaluation. They refer to your child's ability to engage in the normal tasks of daily living and how well he can perform in comparison to others his own age.

The majority of children with AD have an average or higher than average IQ and thus are not likely to be misdiagnosed as MR. The deficits in self-help skills seen in MR are more widespread and the overall functioning is far below the child's age. While children with AD do have deficits in self-help skills, they are quite scattered, with remarkable abilities in some areas and surprisingly limited skills in others. While most children with AD do not have MR, 75–80 percent of children with the other four types of PDD are also diagnosed with MR.

What is Schizoid Personality Disorder?

A personality disorder includes a long-standing pattern of problems in perceiving, relating, and thinking about others and oneself. We all have less-than-desirable aspects to our personalities, but when those aspects become inflexible and cause significant problems in personal, social, and occupational functioning, they are considered to be a disorder. Schizoid Personality Disorder (Schizoid PD) is characterized by severe problems in relating to others. Its symptoms include:

- Lack of desire for close relationships
- Detachment from emotions
- Lack of empathy
- Solitary lifestyle
- Detachment from others
- Limited ability to experience pleasure in activities

These symptoms are very similar to those of AD, making it difficult to separate the two disorders. AD has more prominent and restricted patterns of interest and more observable deficits when interacting with others. The other distinction is that while individuals with Schizoid PD have little desire for friends, those with AD want friends and suffer feelings of loneliness.

Typically, children are not diagnosed with personality disorders, thus it would be unusual to have your child diagnosed with Schizoid PD. However adolescents, and more commonly, adults with AD might be diagnosed with Schizoid PD. Some researchers think that AD and Schizoid PD might actually be one in the same.

What is Reactive Attachment Disorder?

Reactive Attachment Disorder (RAD) involves severely disturbed social relatedness that starts before the age of five years. The child fails to respond to people in an appropriate way, either being excessively withdrawn (inhibited type) or indiscriminately overly affectionate with many people (disinhibited type), some of whom are strangers. This disorder most often occurs in children who lack the opportunity to bond to a parent or caretaker, such as children who live in multiple foster care situations or are raised by severely abusive and/or neglectful parents.

AD is not likely to be mistaken for the disinhibited type of RAD, as AD children are not inappropriately affectionate. However, AD and the inhibited type of RAD both share oddities in their level of interest in interacting with others. Determining if the social deficits of poor eye contact, lack of empathy, and limited ability to share in the interests and joy of others is due to AD or RAD can present a challenge. The history of the emotional attachments the child has can be a distinguishing determinant, with AD children generally having bonds with supportive parents. The AD child also has problems with communication and restricted patterns of interest that are absent in RAD.

What is Sensory Integration Disorder?

Sensory Integration Disorder (SID) is a relatively newly defined complex disorder of the brain. Although not included in the *DSM-IV-TR* and lacking specific symptoms and criteria for diagnosis, it is recognized by many professionals.

Children with SID either are excessively overreactive to stimulation and shrink away from it, as is the case in AD, or are quite the opposite, with a limited responsiveness and a consequent seeking of stimulation, as may also be seen in children with ADHD. Which type of stimulation is upsetting and which is favored by these children varies from child to child. Their abnormal response to stimulation can lead to problems in daily life due to their emotional and behavioral intensity. Many children with AD have intense reactions to stimulation. They may be:

- Overly sensitive to light
- Stiff and avoidant of touch
- Distressed by motion
- Upset by noise
- Irritated by tags, elastic, seams, and textures in clothes
- Picky with textures in food

Extreme reactions that seem to come out of nowhere are commonly seen in children with AD. Usually these seemingly unprovoked reactions can be traced to some irritating stimulation that the child is unable to tell you about. Children with SID are treated by occupational therapists to help them overcome and cope with their extreme sensitivities.

What is Developmental Coordination Disorder?

Developmental Coordination Disorder (DCD) is a childhood disorder characterized by poor coordination and clumsiness. Children with DCD have marked difficulties with gross and/or fine motor movement that interfere with their academic performance and/or daily life activities. Roughly 6 percent of school-age children have some degree of Developmental Coordination Disorder. Children with DCD may trip over their own feet, run into other children, have trouble holding objects, and have an unsteady gait, similar to the clumsiness seen in children with AD.

Developmental Coordination Disorder may appear in conjunction with other learning disorders or it may occur alone. Communication Disorders and Disorder of Written Expression are two of the learning disorders often associated with this condition. Children with AD are often poorly coordinated, some severe enough to be diagnosed with DCD.

Children with DCD are identified by parents and teachers as clumsy, awkward, and poor in athletics. Fine motor skills such as writing and buttoning clothing can be a challenge for these children. Gross motor skills like running, hopping, kicking a ball, riding a bike, skating, and catching a ball may be noticeably delayed. Children are diagnosed with DCD if they fall below expectations for their age in these types of skills.

Writing can be one of the most frustrating challenges. Children with fine motor problems write extremely large, very messy, cannot write on a line, and have many erasures to the point of tearing the paper. Their frustration can result in avoiding school and homework, crying, and arguments about having to write. Children with DCD can suffer related emotional problems due to their physical limitations. They avoid difficult tasks and activities with procrastination, refusal, or tantrums. Their behavior problems may overshadow their motor problems, and diagnosis of DCD can easily be missed.

Gross motor problems tend to interfere with self-esteem and social relationships more than academic abilities. Children who are clumsy and uncoordinated are easily observed on the playground by their peers, who reject them when it comes time to pick teammates for games. Embarrassment, frustration, and anger can result in these children engaging in inappropriate behaviors, including starting arguments, grabbing the ball in order to get attention, physical fights, and socially isolating themselves as they try to escape peer rejection and ridicule.

DCD is diagnosed and treated by occupational therapists, often provided by the public school special education services.

What is a communication disorder?

Communication disorders are disorders of speech and language. The various types of communication disorders range from simple sound substitutions to the inability to understand or use language. Odd language is part of AD, therefore evaluation by a speech pathologist is essential. Some children with AD will have both the odd use of language as part of AD and an additional communication disorder.

Expressive Language Disorders manifest in difficulties producing speech sounds, inappropriate use of sounds or words, stuttering, poor articulation, or problems with pitch, volume, or voice quality. Many of these are characteristic of AD. Children who have trouble understanding words and sentences are diagnosed with Mixed Receptive-Expressive Language Disorder.

Communication disorders are evaluated, diagnosed, and treated by speech pathologists, specialists with a master's degree and license to practice speech therapy. Public schools provide speech therapy through their special education programs. While children with AD and/or communication disorders may qualify for the therapy, most speech pathologists agree that the limited amount of speech therapy provided by public schools is usually insufficient, and parents may therefore want to seek additional speech therapy from a private speech pathologist.

Problems of mood and self-esteem can result from communication disorders as children may be teased and rejected by their peers.

What is a learning disorder?

Learning disorders (LD) occur when a child's academic achievement in a specific subject is significantly below what would be expected for their age, school experience, and intellectual ability. Learning disorders can occur in reading, mathematics, and writing, with reading accounting for about 80 percent. LD are not obvious, and without proper evaluation, they can easily be overlooked. A review of the child's report cards and annual academic achievement test scores are a good first step in discovering if a learning disorder exists. A child who has one or more academic areas significantly below his other areas may have a learning disorder. Learning disorders are present in all levels of intelligence. A child with a learning disorder may be gifted, average, or even below average. Because learning disorders are common in children with AD, it is important that your child be evaluated.

To determine if a child has a learning disorder, she must undergo standardized academic achievement testing to assess what age level and grade level of learning she has achieved. An IQ test must also be given in order to assess the child's intellectual capabilities. Generally, if the child has a significant difference between academic achievement and IQ, a learning disorder is diagnosed. Children with AD and LD may have deficits in specific cognitive functions such as memory, auditory processing, visual processing, and attention, among others.

Reading disorders, which have also been called dyslexia, manifest in impairments of reading accuracy, speed, or comprehension. Mathematics disorders are displayed by impairment in mathematical calculation or mathematical reasoning. Written Expression Disorder is manifested by impairment in the ability to compose written text due to trouble with punctuation, grammar, organization, spelling, and excessively poor handwriting.

Learning disorders are treated with special education and educational therapy. Some children with a learning disorder remain in the mainstream classroom full time. Others stay mainstreamed but have resource services for one or more hours per week where they are placed with a special education teacher who helps them learn techniques to compensate for their specific learning disorder. More severely learning-disordered children may be placed in a full-time special education classroom or go to a private school that specializes in learning disorders.

What is Social Phobia?

Social Phobia, also called Social Anxiety Disorder, is a significant fear of social situations in which the person might be embarrassed. People with Social Phobia are excessively worried about being judged, humiliated, and ridiculed by others. Individuals with Social Phobia have poor social skills. They are hypersensitive to criticism and have low self-esteem. They are uncomfortable making eye contact, initiating conversations, and speaking in front of others. While adults are able to recognize what is causing them to feel anxious, children typically are not able to do so. Children with Social Phobia may back away from interacting with others, avoid playing in a group, stay on the outside of group activities, and prefer to interact with familiar adults. Their chronic avoidance of interacting with peers deprives them of the normal opportunities to learn social skills from experience. Thus, as children with Social Phobia grow older, they become increasingly anxious due to the failure to develop appropriate ways to interact with age-mates.

Social Phobia lacks the restricted interest patterns, insistence on routine, and odd use of language that is seen in AD. However, many of the symptoms of social phobia are displayed by children with AD, making it difficult to distinguish between the two disorders.

What is Tourette's Disorder?

Tourette's is a disorder of multiple tics, including motor and vocal tics that are present for more than one year. A tic is a sudden, rapid, involuntary, and recurrent stereotyped movement or vocalization. Tics are experienced as being irresistible but can be suppressed for varying lengths of time, especially during periods of interesting activities. Alternatively, they can be increased by stress. Examples of Simple Motor Tics include eye blinking, facial grimacing, coughing, shoulder shrugging, and neck jerking. Complex Motor Tics may include facial gestures and touching or smelling an object. Simple Vocal Tics may include sniffing, snorting, barking, throat clearing, and grunting. Complex Vocal Tics include repeating words or phrases out of context, swearing, and repeating the last word or phrase heard.

The frequency and type of tics present in Tourette's changes over time. Most often Tourette's begins with a simple tic of eye blinking. Tics may disappear for periods of time, leading one to think he no longer has it. The same tic may return, or new types of tics may take its place.

Tourette's most commonly starts in childhood and is strongly associated with hyperactivity, distractibility, and impulsivity. It can also be exacerbated by central nervous system stimulant medication, which is commonly given for ADD and ADHD.

Although they can exist together, we do not know how many children with AD have Tourette's Disorder. We do know that it in the general population it is seen in approximately 4–5 individuals per 10,000. It is 1½ to 3 times more common in males than females. It can start as early as age two, but more commonly starts in childhood or adolescence. Once the tics surface, they usually last a lifetime. It is most often a genetic disorder, with only 10 percent of those afflicted having the nongenetic type.

Depression, anxiety, low self-esteem, and embarrassment are also experienced by children with Tourette's. School functioning can also be impaired by the obsessions and compulsions that often coexist with Tourette's.

While neuroleptic medication is the only form of treatment for tics, most physicians avoid prescribing this major tranquilizing drug, preferring instead to let the tics occur naturally.

What are Enuresis and Encopresis?

Enuresis is a disorder of wetting the bed or clothing. As with many developmental disorders, it is not unusual to find enuresis coexisting with AD. Primary enuresis is found in children who have never been dry for longer than six months. Secondary enuresis occurs in children who have achieved dryness for at least six months and then begin to wet themselves. Nocturnal enuresis is more commonly known as bedwetting, while diurnal enuresis occurs during the waking hours. Encopresis involves bowel movements outside the toilet in children age four or older. This is far less common in all children, including those with AD.

Children and teens understandably do not like to admit to toileting problems, and therefore we do not know the number of children and teens with enuresis and encopresis. Studies estimate that at age five years enuresis affects 5–10 percent of all children, with the majority being boys. The incidence drops significantly with age. By age ten, it affects 3 percent of boys and 2 percent of girls. About 1 percent of adolescents still experience enuresis. Encopresis is present in only 1 percent of five-year-olds and, as with enuresis, is more common in boys. Enuresis has very strong family ties, with 75 percent of those affected having a first-degree biological relative who also had the disorder.

Children eventually outgrow enuresis and encopresis even without treatment. However, years of frustration between parent and child can have a very negative effect on the relationship and the child's self-esteem. Having enuresis or encopresis is associated with a higher incidence of coexisting behavioral symptoms. Many children who bedwet avoid sleepovers and overnight camps due to fear of being discovered by their peers as a bedwetter, which typically results in devastating ridicule and humiliation that is difficult to overcome even after the problem no longer exists.

The emotional consequences of enuresis and encopresis make treatment necessary. However, no psychotherapy should be started until medical clearance is obtained by a pediatric urologist and/or gastroenterologist who can ensure there are no physical causes to the wetting or soiling. If physical causes are ruled out, emotional causes need to be considered. Anxiety, changes in the family, and emotional trauma are commonly seen in children with secondary enuresis and encopresis.

What is a nonverbal learning disorder?

Although this disorder is not listed in the *DSM-IV-TR*, it is gaining increasing recognition. It is thought that 1–10 percent of children with learning disorders have NVLD, which affects girls as often as boys. It is believed to be a neurophysiologic disorder originating in the right hemisphere of the brain, the portion of the brain that processes nonverbal information. Some children with NVLD have brain scans that show mild abnormalities of the right cerebral hemisphere. Many have a history of head injury, radiation treatments on the head, treatment for hydrocephalus, or brain tissue removed from their right hemisphere. However, many children with NVLD have no such history and are found to have normal brain scans.

Unlike other learning disorders that can be measured with standardized testing, NVLD is based upon a group of symptoms that together form a disorder. The cluster of symptoms is varied and impacts motor skills, visual-spatial skills, and social skills—the very skills affected by AD.

NVLD causes impairment both academically and socially. These children usually have good vocabulary, memory, and verbal skills. They read well, but because they focus excessively on details, they fail to understand the bigger picture. Information is understood at a concrete level, and they miss out on abstract concepts.

The child with NVLD commonly appears awkward and is poorly coordinated in both fine and gross motor skills. She may have difficulty learning to ride a bike or kick a soccer ball. Fine motor skills, such as cutting with scissors or tying shoelaces, are delayed.

In the social arena, children with NVLD miss the nuances of interactions as they fail to recognize nonverbal behavior of body language, facial expression, and tone of voice. They do not adjust to changes easily, may be fearful of new situations, and lack common sense. They are unable to look and learn and generalize from one situation to another. They do not perceive subtle cues in the environment such as when something has gone far enough; the idea of personal space; the facial expressions of others; or when another person is registering pleasure or displeasure. All these symptoms result in difficulty making and keeping friends, which in turn can cause anxiety, depression, and low self-esteem.

These symptoms are all the symptoms of AD, and there exists a current debate as to whether or not these are actually two different disorders or one disorder with two different names.

What is Semantic Pragmatic Disorder?

Semantic Pragmatic Disorder is not a formally recognized disorder in the *DSM IV TR*, and some researchers question its existence. However, speech therapists use it to describe individuals who have difficulty with how they use language. Semantics refer to the meaning of words, while pragmatics refer to how words are used in context. Individuals who are labeled as having this disorder have a near-normal vocabulary, use grammar appropriately, and have normal pronunciation. Their language problems lie in having difficulty with:

- Initiating conversation
- Sustaining conversation
- Shifting from topic to topic in conversation
- Using words out of context

Because it is unusual to find these types of language problems in the absence of a behavioral, emotional, or cognitive disorder, if your child has been identified as having Semantic Pragmatic Disorder or any speech or language impairment, it is important that she be evaluated by a child psychologist to determine if she also has a psychological or developmental disorder. When language problems interfere with basic conversation skills, social relationship difficulties automatically follow, sometimes making it difficult to determine if the language problems caused the social problems, or if the language problems are just a symptom of a more serious disorder.

What is Gifted and Twice Exceptional?

Being gifted is certainly not a disorder, nor is it even a formal classification. Schools often use the term gifted to refer to students who have superior intelligence. Many children with AD are also identified as gifted. They have superior intelligence, particularly verbal intelligence, and excellent long-memory capabilities.

Decades ago, children accepted into the Gifted and Talented Education program, commonly called GATE, were not only superior intellectually, but they were creative, had excellent social skills, and were free of behavior problems. They truly seemed to be given the gift of overall superior functioning. Over the years, as more and more highly intelligent children were found to have coexisting psychological disorders, the definition of gifted has narrowed. Currently, if your child has an IQ of 130 or greater on a standardized IQ, he probably qualifies as gifted regardless of how many disorders and social and behavioral problems he has. These intelligent and psychologically disordered children have given birth to the relatively new term twice exceptional. Children who are highly intelligent and have ADHD or AD are the most common twice-exceptional student. Smart as a whip but behaviorally, emotionally, and socially challenging to teachers and peers, these children are spurring a whole new field of research.

Chapter 4

SOCIAL SKILLS

- What are the social skills problems seen in Asperger's Disorder?
- How are social skills displayed by the elementary school child with Asperger's Disorder?
- How are social skills displayed by the middle school teen with Asperger's Disorder?
- How are social skills displayed by the high school teen with Asperger's Disorder?
- What are the negative effects of poor social skills?
- What is the normal development of friendships?
- How do children with Asperger's Disorder develop friendships?
- Are children and teens with Asperger's Disorder interested in having friends?
- What is experience sharing?
- How do children with Asperger's Disorder experience share?
- How can I help my child with experience sharing?
- What are social referencing and coregulation?
- How do children and teens with Asperger's Disorder do with social referencing and coregulation?
- How can I help my child with social referencing and coregulation?
- What is social maintenance and repair?
- How do children and teens with Asperger's Disorder do with social maintenance and repair?
- How can I help my child with social maintenance and repair?
- What is social-emotional expression?
- How do children and teens with Asperger's Disorder do with social-emotional expression?
- What is social skills therapy?
- What should I look for in social skills therapy?
- What are storyboards?
- What are behavior bubbles?
- How can I use behavior bubbles to help my child?
- How can I teach my child to recover from social faux pas?
- How can movies help my child with social skills?
- How can a club help my child with social skills?
- What social skills should I work on with my child?
- How can my child's teacher help her function better in a group?
- What can schools do to protect children with Asperger's Disorder from bullying?

What are the social skills problems seen in Asperger's Disorder?

Having AD guarantees trouble interacting with others. Every symptom of AD makes it difficult for the AD child to be accepted by others. Not only do his peers not like him, his teachers, older schoolmates, and adults also do not find him pleasurable to be around. He is out of sync with the social dances of talking, playing, sharing, taking turns, and showing mutual interest and excitement that are part of friendship. AD children do not:

- Make consistent eye contact when talking, listening, or playing
- Notice, read, or understand social cues and body language
- Experience or show interest in other people
- Experience or display empathy
- Share in the interests and achievements of others
- Participate in the give and take of relationships, conversations, and play

While these characteristics might make the AD child appear cold and uncaring, this is not the case. It is not that he has chosen not to care about others; it is that it never enters his mind to consider the other person. The way he interacts with others seems right to him, and he is oblivious to his blatant social mistakes that others see so easily.

Social Skills Difficulties of AD Children and Teens

Problems with Play	*Problems with Friendships*	*Problems with Conversing*
Little imaginative play	Poor eye contact	Monopolizes
Poor cooperative play	Little interest in others	Off-topic
Dominates play	Lacks empathy	Cannot read social cues
Wants complete control of the play	Egocentric	Limited use of gestures
Insists others play exactly their way	May prefer to be alone	Monotone voice
Trouble with group play	Fails to complement peers	Advanced vocabulary
Invades others' personal space	Cannot function in a group	Limited facial expressions
Plays alongside but not with peers	Lacks common social sense	Trouble joining conversations
Uses playmates as objects	Oblivious to social feedback	Bland emotional expression
Trouble joining a group in play	Better with younger children	Dominates conversation
Difficulty sharing toys and games	Better with adults	Limited range of topics
Poor sportsmanship	Emotionally detached	Lectures rather than converses

Social Skills Difficulties of AD Children and Teens continued

Problems with Play	Problems with Friendships	Problems with Conversing
Repetitive organizing of toys	Does not repair conflicts	Loud volume
May prefer to play alone	Does not accept others' views	
Limited pretend or thematic play	Cannot tolerate criticism	
Lacks flexibility in play	Does not initiate contact	
Ritualistic play	Does not express joy easily	
Rigidly follows rules of games	Limited shared enjoyment	
Limited play interests		
Quick to expel peers from play		

How are social skills displayed by the elementary school child with Asperger's Disorder?

In hindsight, many parents report that social problems began to surface in preschool. Those early signs become more apparent in elementary school. AD children will either be withdrawn from social interactions, preferring to stay by themselves, or quite the opposite, where they are intrusive, loud, relentless, and annoying to their peers. Sadly, their unusual manner of interacting is easy to observe, and their peers quickly avoid them. The failure to develop friendships is often the deciding factor in parents seeking an evaluation.

The AD child cannot sustain friendships, partially due to his rigid insistence of rules and his inflexibility in play. He is strictly bound to the rules and will not forgive cheating by his peers. He tattles on his classmates and is oblivious to the social code of not snitching on your peers. His poor motor skills make him low on the list of playmates for games. His need for sameness may become more apparent and his special interests become more developed. As he becomes more knowledgeable about his special interest, his monologues become longer and he is unable to have reciprocal conversations. His advanced vocabulary and knowledge continue to impress adults but alienates peers who do not understand him.

How are social skills displayed by the middle school teen with Asperger's Disorder?

While others their age are making deeper friendships that involve trust, secrets, and common interests, the AD teen remains socially isolated. The social patterns he displayed in elementary school years continue, and his peers are even less willing to tolerate him. As cliques form at school, the AD adolescent is excluded. Lacking common social sense, the AD teen is at risk of being the brunt of pranks or egged on to act out inappropriate behaviors. He is also a prime candidate for public taunting and ridicule.

Fashion, fads, and trends are often ignored by the AD teen as he pursues his unique special interest. Wanting to have friends, the AD teen is at risk for depression as he becomes increasingly aware with each passing year that he lacks the ability to change his social life. If he can find a peer who shares a similar interest, his middle school years will be far better than the child who is without a friend. Even if the friendship is based primarily on pursuing talk and activities related to their special interest, it can be a significant deterrent to depression.

How are social skills displayed by the high school teen with Asperger's Disorder?

Teens with AD are typically described as socially stiff, awkward, emotionally blunted, self-centered, inflexible, misinterpreting social cues, lacking in common sense, unable to have reciprocal conversations, and unable to understand unspoken messages.

Yet life for the high school teen with AD can sometimes be less painful than earlier years. As his peers gain more social maturity and sensitivity, there is often less teasing in high school. More social opportunities exist within the various interest groups and clubs common to high school campuses.

As the adolescent teen with AD gains more confidence, he will likely reach out to initiate peer interactions. While a positive move, it can also increase his chances of being rejected. Navigating the dating world is difficult for most teens, but it is especially difficult for AD teens. As your adolescent becomes interested in dating, she can be easily confused, not knowing how to tell if the object of her affection is flirting with interest or just being polite. Boys with AD can have great trouble recognizing polite signs of rejection and may pursue contact with girls who thought they made it clear they were not interested. Girls can be vulnerable to being taken advantage of by their male classmates.

What are the negative effects of poor social skills?

The ability to interact, get along, and develop and maintain relationships is a powerful predictor of current as well as later psychological adjustment. Young children with poor social skills are unhappy, are alienated from their peers, have poor achievement levels, and have low self-esteem. Peer rejection in adolescence is even more destructive with increased school failure, absenteeism, dropping out, and delinquency. In adulthood, our social skills play a large role in the type of work we are able to find and whether or not we can maintain it. It determines whether or not we will have friends and romantic partners, and ever marry and raise a family.

Friendships are viewed by most people as a very important part of life. Through friendships, we experience feelings of being liked, valued, admired, cared about, trusted, and loved. With this come feelings of positive self-worth, a sense of belonging, and feelings of worthiness.

The inability to navigate the social world in childhood and adolescence has a profound effect on the social life of adults. Half of adults with AD report having only one or two social activities in any given month. More than 35 percent have absolutely none. These statistics drive home the need for intensive social skills training during childhood and adolescence.

What is the normal development of friendships?

Once children discover cooperative play, they increasingly seek out peers to share in the fun of playing. As young as three, children begin to understand that in order to keep a playmate around, you must take turns, share, and compromise.

Around ages six to nine, the concept of reciprocity and mutuality is present. Friends are chosen based on mutual interests. They develop increasing awareness that their classmates have different viewpoints from their own, and with each year find this to be a valuable contributor to their friendships, as it adds novelty and enrichment. Children also become better at interpreting the emotions and intentions of others and taking the perspective of their friends. They engage in increasing prosocial acts of sharing and helping their peers.

In preteen years, from ages ten to thirteen, friendships involve an increasing exchange of ideas, asking for opinions, and acknowledgment of one another's contribution to the conversation, play, or activity. Friendships at this age are based on common interests and how each can help the other. Children are more careful about what they say and do, knowing it might hurt someone. Friendships last longer at this age and more value is placed on personal attributes of loyalty, trust, and keeping promises.

How do children with Asperger's Disorder develop friendships?

In preschool years, the AD child has little interest in his peers. He does not seek out playmates, preferring to play alone.

In elementary school, the AD child does not experience joint play as fun. He is unable to appreciate that his peers have thoughts, feelings, opinions, and desires different than his own. He cannot engage in the give and take of playing and instead tries to dominate.

In preteen years, the AD child does not appreciate the differences and unique contributions her peers bring to the relationship. She is not interested in what her peers think, feel, or believe. Her interactions are one-sided, and she lacks awareness of how her words and actions might be hurtful to others. As her peers choose friends, share their feelings, and develop trust, the AD teen is still looking for someone to share her special interest. The deeper emotional feelings experienced by teens in friendship eludes the AD adolescent.

While AD children can list what makes a bad friend, they have little idea of what qualities make a good friend. Concepts of trust, loyalty, concern, and devotion to friends escapes their awareness.

Are children and teens with Asperger's Disorder interested in having friends?

Despite their behavior sending signals that they are not interested in friendships, quite the opposite is true. AD children have the same desires as everyone else to have friends. Just like his classmates, the AD child wants to be listened to, cared about, asked to join in playground games, and invited to parties. His wishes, however, usually go unfulfilled, and he suffers from the loneliness that comes from being teased and excluded.

As all children grow older, friendships naturally become deeper, more meaningful, and more important to them. The AD preteen and teen is no different than his age-mates in wanting close friendships. However, he has not gained the social skills to make the stronger bonds he sees his peers forming. The pain of having no one to play with in elementary school becomes more intense in middle school and high school as the AD child has no one to eat lunch with, talk to on the phone, or socialize with on the weekends. In his teen years, his desires for romantic relationships grow just like those of his peers, yet he stands little chance of dating if he has failed to learn social skills.

What is experience sharing?

Social interactions and friendships are shared experiences that involve the interests, thoughts, and emotions of two people. Experience sharing is one of the first social skills infants develop. Besides attachment to a parent, experience sharing is perhaps the most critical social skill necessary for healthy relationships.

Even prior to their first birthday, infants experience share. They point out objects for their parents to see and watch for their parents' reaction. When the parent smiles, the baby smiles too. They are both engaged in the shared experienced of enjoying the object. When the toddler begins to walk, he advances his experience sharing by bringing objects to his parent so that they both can delight in them. As he moves through toddler years, he seeks to experience share with other family members, preschool teachers, and classmates. As he gains more skills, language, interests, and talents, he seeks to share these with others so they each can enjoy them. He also becomes interested in what others have to share with him and takes delight in their happiness. As he grows older, experience sharing continues to form the basis of all his friendships and will do so throughout his life. Those he can experience share with the most will become his closest friends.

How do children with Asperger's Disorder experience share?

AD children do not find pleasure in having a shared experience. Some parents recall that their AD child did not engage in the typical pointing out and bringing of objects during infancy and the toddler years. In preschool, elementary, and later years, the joy and excitement that comes from playing with friends escapes the child with AD. He is not interested in the novelty that a friend or playmate brings to the play experience. Instead, he finds his joy in getting the other person to act out the play exactly as he has it pictured in his mind. He does not want the other child to give input, ideas, or creativity. While other children find that playing, talking, or doing an activity is more fun with someone else, the AD child only likes to have another child around if he can be completely in charge. Play and talking are more enjoyable if they do not have to factor in the wants, needs, interests, and feelings of others. When the AD child does share an item, interest, or thought, he does so to inform rather than to share the experience. When others seek to experience share with him, he shows little response that would motivate the other child to continue the interaction.

How can I help my child with experience sharing?

AD children need to be taught not only *how* to experience share but *why*. The how can be learned through a variety of techniques you will read later in this chapter. The why must come from helping your child learn to enjoy experience sharing. He literally needs to learn that being with others is fun. Most children do not need to be taught this; from infancy through adulthood, we simply feel good in the company of people we like. This pleasure motivates us to seek them out again and again.

Look for moments to express pleasure being in his company, commenting on how it is the shared experience that makes it fun: "I am having so much fun putting on this puppet show with you! It sure beats doing it alone!" Point out positive emotions you see him and his playmate sharing: "Sure looks like you and Joanie are having fun together!"

Place your child in the company of others who enjoy him. Don't worry if this involves more adults than peers. The importance is giving him the experience of bringing pleasure to another person in the hopes that he feels good about it and wants to repeat the experience.

What are social referencing and coregulation?

Social referencing is the observation of emotional reactions in others for the purpose of helping us determine how to respond. When we modify our words or behaviors to more closely match the person we are interacting with, we are engaged in coregulation. Both social referencing and coregulation are essential elements in experience sharing. Successful social interactions and friendships involve each person observing one another and reacting to what the other person has to say, how he feels, what he thinks, and how he behaves. The process is ongoing, where each child shapes what he says and does in reaction to what his friend just said and did.

Social referencing and coregulation are typically done without having to purposely think about it. If our friend is in a great mood and laughing and telling funny stories, we are likely to join him in laughter and maybe even tell some of our own funny stories. There are times, however, when we make a very conscious choice to coregulate in response to our social referencing. If our friend is sad, then we don't laugh and tell jokes even if we are in a good mood. Instead we regulate our words, emotions, and behavior to fit closer to his so he feels comfortable.

How do children and teens with Asperger's Disorder do with social referencing and coregulation?

Children and teens with AD are very poor at social referencing and coregulation.

They do not understand that paying attention to what others are saying, feeling, and doing is an important part of friendships. They lack both the interest and the skill in observing others. They are blind to how others are feeling and are often at a loss as to how to even guess another person's emotion when asked to do so. Regardless of how the other child is feeling and acting, the AD child will simply continue on with whatever thought, word, and emotion he has. This is understandably upsetting to others, who conclude that he is rude and inconsiderate. Most often the AD child simply seems selfish and only interested in what he thinks and wants to do. Yet sometimes his failure to socially reference and coregulate can seem alarmingly insensitive. A peer may want to talk about the death of his pet, to which the AD child responds by talking about his train collection. He does not observe that his friend is sad and without this social reference, he does not coregulate by waiting to talk about trains and instead offer sympathy.

How can I help my child with social referencing and coregulation?

Social referencing and coregulating are difficult social skills for AD children and teens to learn. You can teach your child to socially reference by repeatedly prompting him to notice how the other person is behaving and feeling. Initially, you can be the eyes for your child and interpret for him: "Ken is making faces and gritting his teeth. He seems irritated that you won't share the trucks with him." As you see she is beginning to show signs of social referencing, you can replace your observation with a prompt: "Lindsey, can you tell how Connie is feeling right now since you keep talking and won't let her talk too?" You will have to do social referencing of the mood, thought, behavior, and feelings of others throughout your son or daughter's childhood and adolescent years.

Teaching coregulation can be done at the same time as social referencing. Your child will need to know what to do once you have helped him with the observation. Expect that for many years, you will have to be very specific and direct with him, much like you did when he was a toddler, telling him, "Brandon, you need to listen to Larry."

What is social maintenance and repair?

Friendships take some effort to keep alive. Simple actions of calling friends, inviting them over to play, giving them one of your collector cards, or letting them lick the frosting from the bowl are ways children maintain friendships. Teens may maintain friendships by keeping trust and sharing clothing, music, and secrets. When both friends are equally invested in keeping the friendship alive and each puts forth effort, the better the friendship.

Even equally maintained friendships need occasional repair. Lasting friendships involve both children working to maintain harmony by engaging in experience sharing, social referencing, coregulation, and maintenance. Yet even with both children having good skills, every friendship is bound to have some disagreements and conflicts. Children and teens with good social skills are motivated to repair misunderstandings and resolve conflicts. Good friendships involve both children working to repair the problem.

Friends who share an equal role in maintaining and repairing the friendship are more desirable and more likely to have long-lasting and deeper friendships. If one child has to do all the work to maintain and repair the problems, the friendship is likely to die when he tires of being the only one invested in keeping the friendship alive.

How do children and teens with Asperger's Disorder do with social maintenance and repair?

AD is a great inhibitor to social maintenance and repair. Being friends with an AD child is not likely to be very rewarding. Maintenance of a friendship is not a priority for AD children. They do not understand the concept of extending invitations and creating opportunities for fun as a way to start and maintain a friendship. Nor do they understand that in the midst of interacting with a peer, they must do things to sustain the pleasure if they do not want their playmate to quit and if they hope to have that peer play with them in the future. AD children are focused on their experience, not that of their peer.

Repair is very difficult for AD children. They do not seek to observe how their playmate feels. Nor do they attempt to understand why the other child is upset or what can be done to fix the situation so that they can keep playing together or remain friends. Apologizing for a misunderstanding does not come easy for the AD child. He does not see that he's upset his friend and does not grasp the concept that sometimes you say you are sorry in order to save the friendship.

How can I help my child with social maintenance and repair?

Social maintenance requires that your child work to keep friendships alive. Parents of toddlers and early-elementary children are used to being responsible for their child's social maintenance. As children grow, they become more interested in taking charge of when to initiate contact with their friends and choosing the activities. You will have to keep the job of social maintenance manager far longer than parents of non-AD children. Your child will have more social activities if you take charge of inviting friends over, planning activities and outings that are enticing to her peers, encouraging your child to telephone her friends, and taking her to buy birthday, holiday, get-well, and special-occasion gifts and cards.

Expect to become a social repair expert. Your child will surely have many conflicts with her peers and potential friends. You will have to teach her very directly what she did that upset her friend and what exactly she needs to say and do to try to fix the friendship.

Remembering that it will take years to teach these skills will help you be patient and walk the fine line between giving your child the extra help she needs and being smothering.

What is social-emotional expression?

Children who go out of their way to communicate joy and pleasure during shared activities make more desirable friends than children who do not. When researchers study friendships, they consistently find that the single most important element for children in choosing who they will pick as a friend is that the other child is fun to be around. Teens and adults also like to be around people who are fun. Children and teens that initiate contact with their friends and enthu siastically invite them to engage in fun activities together are viewed as more desirable by their peers.

Clear expression of both positive and negative feelings makes for closer and more emotionally rewarding friendships. For a successful friendship, both children must be interested in how the other person feels. They each must express their feelings and seek to understand what caused the emotions. Clear expression of pleasure can be shared and open display of upset can be discussed and resolved, both of which keep the friendship alive and solid. Children and teens that base their words and actions on the emotional reactions of their friends and playmates are well-liked and sought out by their peers.

How do children and teens with Asperger's Disorder do with social-emotional expression?

Being fun is not commonly regarded as a trait of AD children or teens. They typically have limited emotional engagement with their peers and low emotional expression.

They do not seek to share excitement and do not respond to their peers' indications of pleasure. They do not often approach others and invite them to have fun. Their emotions are typically blunted during play and activities, and whatever joy they experience is hard to detect. If the playmate feels he is the only one having fun, it dampens the overall experience and will probably prevent another invitation to get together. The AD child, however, will report that he had fun and will be left bewildered as to why the peer never invited him to get together again.

Expression of negative emotions is the opposite of how the AD child displays his joy. Anger and frustration are frequently displayed by the AD child, and is often the reason his playmate looks elsewhere for a friend. His expression is likely to be quick to surface, as well as an overreaction to the situation. He will have trouble bringing his upset to closure and moving on.

You will learn more about the emotions of AD individuals and ways you can help your child in chapter 6.

What is social skills therapy?

Social skills therapy (SST) is designed to teach social skills and improve social competence. It is considered to be the primary form of treatment for children and teens with AD. Those who receive SST have a better chance of learning how to have successful social interactions and establish meaningful relationships.

Mental health professionals agree that SST is most successful if it takes place in a group, with peers who have similar social skills deficits. Individual treatment for social skills is not considered an appropriate or effective method. The group setting allows a therapist to observe your child interacting with others and helps him or her provide immediate guidance. It is also the consensus of professionals that SST must be long-term. Because the disorder is lifelong and change is very slow, years of treatment are usually necessary. As with all forms of therapy, the earlier the better.

SST has many benefits over individual therapy for children with AD. It is more cost-effective. It provides a nurturing environment to learn and practice social skills. It provides children and teens with a place to belong and feel accepted by peers. This is also a place where they have a good chance of establishing meaningful friendships with the other group members.

What should I look for in social skills therapy?

While SST programs vary, there are essential elements that you should look for. Be sure to find a long-term program that is a minimum of one year or is ongoing and allows your child to remain in the group for as long as needed. Your child should be placed with children who are similar in functioning level. Many groups will have a mix of children with AD, ADHD, learning disorders, and HFA, all of whom have social skills difficulties. The age of the other group members may vary by two to three years, as therapists tend to match children more by functioning level rather than specific ages. Some groups are mixed with boys and girls, while others are gender-specific. The benefit to a coed group is that it provides your child with the opportunity to interact with both genders. All-girl or all-boy groups can be of benefit in the adolescent years when issues of dating and sexuality surface. Look for a SST program that uses the following techniques to teach social skills:

- Direct instruction
- Role modeling
- Role play
- Positive reinforcement
- Therapist feedback
- Peer feedback
- Peer interaction
- Conversation skills training
- Emotional-expression training
- Social referencing training
- Coregulation training
- Maintenance and repair training

What are storyboards?

Storyboards are miniature picture stories. Using pictures and a few words, storyboards give a script for behavior. They tell a child what behavior is desired, when to do the behavior, and how it affects others. They can be used to remind your child to do a specific behavior.

You can help your child make storyboards with drawings, cartoons, clip art, or magazine pictures, or purchase ready-made pictures and boards called Picture Communication Symbols. Your child will be more likely to work on a particular behavior if she gets to choose which one it is. Work with her to write a script about the behavior. The script should include a positive statement of how the behavior makes others feel good, what the specific behavior is, and several statements about who to use the behavior with and when. If she is able to help choose the words that go on the storyboard, she is more likely to use it. For example, if your child agrees to work on listening to others, her story would be something like this:

- People like it when…
- I listen to them…
- I can listen to…
- My friends when they have something to say…
- I can be quiet and listen to…
- People when they talk…
- I can listen to my teacher…
- I can listen to my mom…
- I can listen to my dad…

Once the story is written, help your child draw or paste simple pictures below the words. For example, a happy face matches the statement "people like it when . . ." and a face with a closed mouth and big ears matches the statement "I listen to . . ."

Short, one-page stories are best. Place the story in a sheet protector and post it in a highly visible place such as your child's desk at school, mirror in the bathroom, or on the front of his notebook.

People Like it When I Say Hi

People 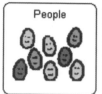	like it	when I say "hi" 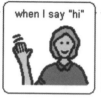	to them.
People 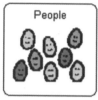	like it 	when I say "hello." 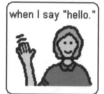	
There are many times 	each day	when "hi" 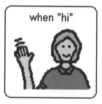	can be good to say.
People 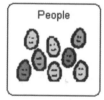	like it	when I say "hi."	
I can say "hi" 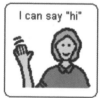	to my mom	when I wake up 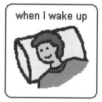	in the morning.
I can say "hi" 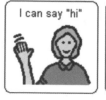	to the bus driver	on the way to school.	

What are behavior bubbles?

Similar to storyboards, behavior bubbles are a tool to help children and teens understand the cause and effect between thoughts and feelings, and words and behavior. As your child begins to understand that what we think causes our feelings, and our feelings lead to our words and behavior, he can begin to make better choices about what he says and does.

A series of simple bubbles are used to fill in thoughts, feelings, words, and actions. You can use behavior bubbles to review a negative situation that happened earlier in the day or week. One set of bubbles is filled in with what actually happened. The second set is used to fill in more positive choices your child could have made.

Help your child fill in the first set with what he was thinking during the situation, what feelings he had, what words he said, what behaviors he did, and what the consequence was. The next step is to help your child fill in the second set of bubbles with better alternatives. What thoughts could he have had that might have been more socially acceptable? What feelings would these thoughts have led to and what would your child have said and done if he had thought differently about the situation? What would the consequence be if he could have done it this way?

How can I use behavior bubbles to help my child?

Behavior bubbles are easy to create. You can make up the behavior bubbles ahead of time, or make it a fun activity where your child chooses the paper and markers and decides who will draw the bubbles and who will do the writing.

Choose a time when your child is calm and no longer upset by the situation. Discuss with your child what happened. Let her tell or write what she was thinking and feeling and what she said and did. Don't worry about spelling and neatness and resist the temptation to

What Happened:	What Would Have Been Better:
THOUGHTS	**THOUGHTS**

Isabella is reaching for my lunch. She is going to steal it from me.

I wonder what Isabella is doing reaching toward my lunch.

I should ask her what she is doing.

| **FEELINGS** | **FEELINGS** |

I am mad!

I am worried she is going to take my lunch.

| **WORDS** | **WORDS** |

I told Isabella, "I hate you! You better leave my lunch alone or I will hit you!"

I ask Isabella, "Isabella, what are you doing?"

| **BEHAVIOR** | **BEHAVIOR** |

I hit Isabella.

I wait to listen to what Isabella says and watch what she does. If she takes my lunch, I ask for it back. If she won't give it back, I will tell the teacher.

talk about why her thoughts, feelings, words, or actions were wrong. The goal is for your child to have an accepting and nurturing environment to express herself without being punished or lectured.

Ask your child what she thinks went wrong in the situation. Be a good listener and be understanding. Ask her if there was another way to think about the situation. If she cannot think of an alternative viewpoint, you can suggest one. Ask her if she had this different thought what feelings she would have had. Then discuss what she would have said and done if she had these different thoughts and feelings. Finally, discuss what the consequence would have been.

How can I teach my child to recover from social faux pas?

Your child will fare better with adults and peers if he learns to recognize when he has made errors in behavior and social interaction. He must then learn how to fix the situation. You can teach him simple statements he can use to show others he knows he made an error and that he is sorry for having done so. Adults and children alike are far more tolerant of people who apologize for their mistakes than those who deny, rationalize, and blame others. AD children and teens have particular difficulty in admitting wrongdoing and apologizing.

Teaching your child the following statements can help your child get out of a negative situation and prevent additional problems:

- I'm sorry.
- I'm sorry; I was not thinking.
- I'm sorry; I did not mean to cause a problem.
- I'm sorry; I did not mean to hurt your feelings.
- I'm sorry; I'm confused. Can we start over?
- I'm sorry; I wasn't paying attention. Can you tell me again?
- I'm sorry; that was the wrong thing for me to say.
- I'm sorry; I don't know what you want me to do.

How can movies help my child with social skills?

Movies are about relationships. The movies many children enjoy are those where the characters are socially clumsy and make blatant social blunders that make the audience laugh. By watching movies, AD children have a fun opportunity to see characters make social mistakes that the AD child can easily identify as wrong. Some of the shows have a costar whose job it is to help a socially deficient character learn what he is doing wrong and teach him the correct social behavior. Be sure to match the movie rating with your child's age and maturity level. You may want to view the movie alone first to determine if it is appropriate for your child. Some fun movies and television shows with great social skills blunders include:

- *Toy Story* (G)
- *Jimmy Neutron Boy Genius* (G)
- *Polar Express* (G)
- *Adventures of Elmo in Grouch Land* (G)
- *Shrek* (G)
- *Willie Wonka and the Chocolate Factory*—1971 version (G)
- *Charlie and the Chocolate Factory* (G)

- *That's So Raven* (TV-G)
- *Third Rock from the Sun* (Not Rated TV series)
- *Mork and Mindy* (Not Rated TV Series)
- *Mr. Bean* (PG)
- *Bicentennial Man* (PG)
- *My Stepmother Is an Alien* (PG)
- *Starman* (PG)
- *Encino Man* (PG)
- *Mean Girls* (PG-13)
- *Billy Madison* (PG-13)
- *The Cable Guy* (PG-13)
- *Ace Ventura: Pet Detective* (PG-13)

Let your child talk as much as she wants, and join her in the comedy and the pointing out of the outlandish blunders. Make your comments fun and lighthearted; you don't want to turn a fun movie experience into a classroom lecture. Simple statements of "Oh my! I can't believe he did that!" or "Wow! Did you see that?" are all that are needed. Do not teach, discuss, or point out how your child's behavior is similar to the characters. Just watch, laugh, and have fun.

How can a club help my child with social skills?

Many children are simply kinder to others outside the school setting, and your child may find more acceptance in an off-campus club. He can join a club for children or teens where he can share similar interests. Some AD children will do well in child-centered clubs; however, many will still be the rejected child and the club is simply one more place for him to feel that he does not belong. A way to avoid this is to join a parent-child club with your child. She will experience a social activity with the safety of your supervision. Plus, the quality time with you will help build lasting bonds. Campfire USA,

Scouts, and Indian Guides/Princess are fantastic opportunities for a rich social life that your child likely cannot initiate and maintain on his own. Volunteer work that you and your child can do together will give him time with you and help him learn charity to others, and give him positive feelings about himself for having been helpful to people in need. A family summer camp where the entire family goes can allow your child the socialization, fun, and freedom camp offers with your eye close by.

What social skills should I work on with my child?

Each child is unique and will have skills he learns naturally and others he does not even know he is supposed to do. You can identify what skills your child does well and which ones he needs to improve upon by simply observing him in various situations with various people. Make a list of how he interacts with his classmates, teachers, coaches, relatives, neighbors, siblings, and parents. You can use the chart to keep track of his strengths and weaknesses. Praise him when he uses proper social skills so you can reinforce his use.

Rate your child on the following social skills by putting a + next to the skills he does well and a - next to those he rarely does and/or does poorly. Use this list to periodically monitor his progress.

Social Skills Chart

	Greeting others		Giving suggestions for play
	Saying goodbye		Accepting suggestions
	Starting a conversation		Asking nicely for help
	Joining a conversation		Accepting help from others
	Maintaining a conversation		Noticing who needs help
	Ending a conversation		Giving appropriate help
	Asking others to play		Resolving conflicts
	Joining existing play		Keeping peers' secrets
	Turning down offers to play		Encouraging others
	Cooperating with game rules		Avoiding negative peers
	Accepting losing at games		Conversing on topic
	Sharing items		Changing topics
	Giving compliments		Compromising
	Accepting compliments		Modifying to fit situation
	Listening to others		Observing social cues
	Expressing emotions		Responding to social cues
	Letting others participate		Avoiding hurt feelings
	Avoiding interrupting		Apologizing
	Accepting when interrupted		Accepting apologies
	Accepting own mistakes		Comforting others
	Accepting others' mistakes		Avoiding criticizing others
	Giving helpful feedback		Playing cooperatively
	Tolerating helpful feedback		Considering others' wishes
	Waiting turn to talk		Keeping promises
	Looking others in the eye		Expressing joy

How can my child's teacher help her function better in a group?

Functioning in groups is one of the more difficult experiences for children with AD. When a teacher instructs students to pick their own teams, the AD child is sure to be the last picked. When teachers direct students to pair up to work on a project or form a group, the AD child is never chosen and the one child who was not fast enough to find a partner ends up "stuck" with the AD child.

Teachers with an AD child in the classroom can be sensitive and reduce the number of times the AD child is rejected, isolated, teased, or excluded by modifying how they create group activities. Instead of letting team captains pick the teams, the teacher can divide the class into teams by various categories (e.g., birthdays between January and June on team A and July through December on team B, names staring with A–L on team A and M–Z on team B, etc.). Instead of leaving children to form their own pairs, teachers can be creative in the way they form groups (e.g., putting raffle tickets in a jar and having each student pick one and find the other student with the same number). Your child's teacher may appreciate your creative ideas on how to help your child avoid being excluded by his peers.

What can schools do to protect children with Asperger's Disorder from bullying?

Disability harassment is a form of discrimination prohibited by Section 504 of the 1973 Rehabilitation Act and Title II of the Americans with Disabilities Act of 1990. Students cannot learn in an atmosphere of fear, intimidation, or ridicule. Each school has a legal obligation to prevent and respond to disability harassment. Your child's school should have a clear policy that states bullying is unacceptable and violates federal law, as well as have written action and grievance procedures.

In order to meet the legal standard of harassment, the U.S. Department of Education specifies that it must be identified as "intimidation or abusive behavior towards a student with a disability that creates a hostile environment by interfering with or denying a student's participation in or receipt of benefits, services, or opportunities in the institution's program." The harassment must be severe enough to interfere with your child being able to benefit from the Free and Appropriate Education that he is legally entitled to. Typical teasing common to most children does not meet the standard.

Examples of a hostile environment would include a child who is bullied and pretends to be sick so he can avoid school, a student who stops using his laptop in class as an accommodation tool because the teacher criticizes her in front of her classmates, or a student who is repeatedly called names in class by his peers, resulting in outbursts that stop him from being able to participate in classroom lessons.

If your child is being harassed by either students or school personnel, write to her school and request an investigation and that steps be taken to prevent any further harassment. If your school fails to comply, you have the right to file a complaint with your local school board under due process.

Chapter 5

THINKING PATTERNS

- What are the thinking problems of Asperger's Disorder?
- What is Theory of Mind?
- What is the impact of a poor Theory of Mind?
- How is Theory of Mind measured?
- How is Theory of Mind measured in older children and teens?
- Why is Theory of Mind so important?
- What is the normal development of Theory of Mind?
- Can children with Asperger's Disorder be taught Theory of Mind?
- How can I use games to help my child learn Theory of Mind?
- What is literal interpretation?
- How can I help my child with literal interpretation?
- What is black-and-white thinking?
- How can I help my child with black-and-white thinking?
- What is rule-bound thinking?
- How can I help my child with rule-bound thinking?
- What is truth-bound thinking?
- How can I help my child with truth-bound thinking?
- What is perfectionistic thinking?
- How can I help my child with perfectionistic thinking?
- What is catastrophic thinking?
- How can I help my child with catastrophic thinking?
- What is rigid thinking?
- How can I help my child with rigid thinking?
- What is perseverative thinking?
- How can I help my child with perseverative thinking?
- What is generalization?
- How can I help my child with generalization?

What are the thinking problems of Asperger's Disorder?

If we had to choose one characteristic of AD that is the most problematic, it would likely be problems in thinking. The deficiencies in thinking have little to do with thinking in terms of being smart or having the ability to learn. Instead they are related to the way children with AD think about people, social interactions, and relationships.

AD individuals have no trouble thinking about how things work, but great difficulty understanding how people work. The thinking problems seen in AD include:

- Unawareness of others' feelings
- Inability to read other people's intentions
- Inability to see another person's perspective
- Inability to tell what others are thinking
- Interpreting others' words literally
- Viewing things in black-and-white
- Rule-bound thinking
- Perfectionistic thinking
- Catastrophic thinking
- Rigid thinking
- Perseverative thinking
- Failure to generalize

What is Theory of Mind?

Theory of Mind is the ability to make attributions. Attributions are the thoughts we create about others in order to explain what happens in our interactions with and observations of them. No one actually teaches us to make attributions; we just do it automatically. For the most part, we can make good guesses at someone's intentions.

From these inferences, we determine how to react to them. AD children, however, do not know how to make attributions. This is because they are deficient in Theory of Mind (ToM).

The concept of Theory of Mind has also been labeled as mind blindness, mentalizing, and mind reading. Each of these terms defines the ability to infer what others are thinking, feeling, believing, and desiring, and what their intentions and motivations are. Using ToM, we can make sense of what people say and do and predict what they will do next. In essence, we can stand inside someone else's shoes. Using ToM gives us an understanding of others that allows us to guide our behavior and interactions with them.

Children and teens with AD are deficient in ToM. They do not comprehend that others have thoughts and feelings that are different from their own. They cannot stand in someone else's shoes.

What is the impact of a poor Theory of Mind?

Problems with ToM can have a significant negative impact on the social interactions and relationships of children and teens with AD. Virtually every social encounter requires the use of ToM. Because he lacks this ability, your child may make countless social errors every day, as he says and does what he wants without consideration for its impact on others.

Without ToM, the AD child is not able to determine how someone else feels. His inability to read emotional expression in the eyes and face results in insensitivity to others. He will be perceived as rude, uncaring, and disrespectful, although this is not his intention. He cannot decipher intentions and therefore often misinterprets the reasons behind people's actions. Being unable to distinguish between accidental and intentional actions, the AD child can seem almost paranoid, as he usually assumes others are against him. Not being able to consider someone's feelings, the AD child is blunt to the point of insulting. When conflicts occur, the AD child cannot see the other person's side and will rigidly insist he is right. He will not repair relationships with an apology because he does recognize that his peer is upset. These repeated social errors cause rejection by peers. Fortunately, there are ways to help your child learn ToM that you will learn later in this book.

How is Theory of Mind measured?

There are no formal tests to measure or diagnose ToM. However, there are several techniques that can give your child's evaluator an idea of the level of ToM your child has developed. One such technique is the Smarties task. In the Smarties task, the child is shown a container of Smarties candies, or another type of highly recognized candy container. The child is asked what is inside the container, with the expected answer to be "Smarties candies." The examiner opens the container and instead of Smarties, coins come out. The child is then told that their mother is going to be shown the Smarties container and the child is asked what she thinks her mother will say. Children who have ToM say their mother will guess that the container has Smarties in it. Children without ToM will say their mother will say the container has coins in it. AD children do not understand that their mother does not know the examiner has played a trick and put coins in the container instead of the candy. They do not understand the difference between what they know and what the other person knows.

How is Theory of Mind measured in older children and teens?

At ages six to twelve, ToM can be assessed using the Strange Stories test. The test begins with simple stories of common social situations. For example, to test if a child can understand that his words can hurt people, he is read a story about a boy who hates the gift his parents got him for his birthday yet tells them that he loves it. Most children by age seven understand that this type of white lie is usually acceptable in order to avoid hurting someone's feelings. The AD child at the same age cannot understand why the boy would lie. In this test, the stories become more complex and test more advanced ToM skills such as understanding jokes, pretending, misunderstanding, persuading, figures of speech, irony, forgetting, bluffing, and contradictory emotions. Stories From Everyday Life and ToM Test are two other tools evaluators and therapists may use to measure and monitor progress in your child's ToM abilities.

These tests can be very useful in helping your child's therapist set specific goals for treatment. Periodic readministration of the tests can help measure progress.

Why is Theory of Mind so important?

Virtually every interaction we have with people requires the use of ToM. We connect and relate to others who notice our feelings and comment on them, validate them, and provide us with support. Those who ignore, minimize, or criticize our feelings are usually not invited to remain in our lives. Children and teens who lack ToM have great difficulty making even one friend due to their inability to understand the feelings of others.

We also choose friends with whom we can converse and share ideas. People who disregard what we say, change the subject, and monopolize the conversation are quickly judged to lack the qualities desired for further conversation, let alone a friendship.

The AD child does not recognize when he has hurt someone's feelings and therefore does nothing to repair it. He also fails to learn from his social errors. He lacks awareness that he even did something wrong. Even if told what he said or did that was hurtful, he cannot understand why the other person would feel upset.

Without the ability to think about what others are feeling and thinking, the AD child or teen stands little chance of being included in conversations, play, and activities with peers.

ToM allows each of us to make inferences about others so that we can explain to ourselves their behavior and make predictions about what they will do next.

What is the normal development of Theory of Mind?

ToM develops automatically for most children without formal instruction. Infants as young as nine months can engage in the beginning stages of ToM. By engaging in joint attention, they seek to point out objects to others to share in the delight. A baby points out objects and watches her parents to see if they smile, thus showing her that they enjoy it too. Failure to point out objects and have a shared experience of pleasure is one of the first indicators of AD and suggests a lack of ToM.

By one and a half years, ToM advances to include pretend play, where a baby can use objects in an imaginary fashion instead of solely for the intended purpose. He can use a cardboard box for his train or a stick for his magic wand. The AD child's failure to develop imaginary play is the next indicator that surfaces. However, often-times it is only in retrospect that parents will recall that their AD child seemed very bound to playing with toys exactly as they were intended to be used and rarely engaged in make-believe.

By the end of the second year, toddlers begin to ask questions about what others are saying, doing, and thinking. While they cannot yet guess what the other person is likely to be thinking, they do understand that others have thoughts and feelings that might be different from theirs. The AD child, on the other hand, does not make these observations about others or question what they are doing or why they are doing it.

At age three, toddlers understand that seeing something leads to knowing about it. They grasp the idea that if someone did not see something happen they won't know it occurred. In contrast, AD toddlers assume everyone knows what they know even if the other person was not there to observe it.

By age four, children begin to develop the ability to guess what another person is thinking. They can guess why another person is engaging in a particular behavior and can guess how someone feels. At this level, they have ToM. AD children do not even think about what others are thinking, feeling, or doing.

As children grow older, they develop increasing complex abilities in ToM. The AD child, however, is seriously delayed and remains stuck at the stage of only considering what he thinks.

Can children with Asperger's Disorder be taught ToM?

Mental health professionals believe that to some degree, children and teens with AD can be taught ToM. Through training in emotions, social skills, and "mind reading," AD children can gain some ability to understand what others are thinking and feeling and use this to guide their words and behavior.

While ToM comes naturally to other children, the AD child must be educated as to what ToM is and why it is important to use it. The AD child actually has to run through a checklist of questions:

1. What is this other person thinking?
2. Why is he doing what he is doing?
3. How is he feeling right now?
4. What is he going to do and say next?
5. How should I respond?

Processing all this takes time for the AD child.

When AD children receive training in ToM, they are found to make fewer social errors. However, the manner in which they use ToM skills is observed to be slow and robotic. It is as if they learn the steps to the dance but have no rhythm.

How can I use games to help my child learn Theory of Mind?

The goal of teaching ToM is to increase your child's ability to understand what other people are thinking and feeling. Developing these skills will improve your child's ability to have empathy for others. Games can be a fun way for your child to learn ToM in a way that he does not approach as a learning experience. A variety of games exist that involve guessing what someone else is thinking. While not designed for the purpose of developing ToM, the following games can give your child direct experience focusing on what the other person is thinking:

- **Password**: Players take turns giving one-word clues while the other player tries to guess the password.
- **I Spy**: Players take turns secretly choosing an object in the room and the other player tries to guess the object.
- **20 Questions**: Players take turns secretly thinking of an item and the other player is allowed twenty questions to guess the item.
- **Would You Rather . . . ?** Players read a card describing a scenario and each player secretly writes down what they would do in the situation. Players earn points if they correctly guess what the other person would do.

What is literal interpretation?

AD children interpret things very literally. They do not understand sarcasm, figures of speech, or even playful teasing. It is as if they only hear the words that people say and are deaf to the tone, blind to the facial expression, and oblivious to the intent.

Their response to what others say can sound disrespectful or smart-mouthed. If you tell your daughter, "I can't stand this anymore!" She may respond with, "Well, then sit down." She is not talking back. She really thinks that you literally do not feel as if you can physically stand up. If your son asks when he will get a television in his room and you tell him, "Oh yeah, that'll happen!" with a roll of your eyes and a sarcastic tone of voice, he will ask you when exactly will he get his television. He hears your words but misses your tone of voice and facial expression. Children with AD have a robotic-like interpretation of words where the emotions are not registered.

How can I help my child with literal interpretation?

Knowing your child does not "read between the lines" will help you to be more empathic and patient and less reactive when he seems to be mocking you. When your child was quite young, you probably were very patient in explaining things to her, telling her something over and over until she got it. Children with AD require this same kind of patience and repetition for years beyond what you would normally expect. Through no fault of their own they simply are extremely slow to understand the meaning of what others say unless it is very obvious and leaves no room for distortion.

You can save your child confusion and embarrassment by interpreting for her. Instead of letting her ask someone where the worms are that the early bird gets, you can interpret this for her in a question as if you are the one who needs help, such as asking, "Do you mean we should get up early to get our chores done before we go to the beach?" You can also phrase the interpretation in the form of an agreement, such as, "That's right—we should get up early so we have the rest of the day to play."

What is black-and-white thinking?

Black-and-white thinking refers to seeing situations in polar opposites. Things are either all one way or all the opposite way. Black-and-white thinking prevents the AD child from seeing shades of gray.

Since situations are usually complex and have many ways in which they can be viewed, the black-and-white thought patterns of the AD child can be incredibly frustrating for others. It is normal to respond with logic and reasoning when your child has his view set in stone. Unfortunately, children and teens with AD do not respond to logic. You are likely to have countless instances where you just gave up, concluding there was simply just no reasoning with your child.

AD children cannot view situations from any perspective other than their own. They do not consider alternative viewpoints. When suggestions are given to try to see things from the other person's perspective, they are at a loss. Because they see only their viewpoint, they are absolutely sure their view is correct. If someone disagrees with him, the AD child becomes very frustrated. He will insist that others accept his viewpoint and he has no interest whatsoever in what the other person has to say.

How can I help my child with black-and-white thinking?

Logic, reasoning, and explanation unfortunately results in the AD child becoming angry and more insistent on his viewpoint. It is better to let him have his viewpoint. When you catch yourself feeling frustrated that he simply won't listen to reason, you need to recognize that he is stuck in black-and-white thinking and end the conversation.

At a later point in time, when he is calm, you can bring up the topic and together make a list of all the possible ways to view the situation or all the possible solutions. Write down all possible ideas regardless of how good they are and do not make negative comments—otherwise your child will become resistant. Write the pros and cons of each one and then discuss which idea looks the best. Through this technique, you are teaching your child how to look at situations from another perspective. He may still rigidly hold to his original idea, but at least you are teaching him how to consider other options.

You can also encourage him to think about what someone else would do if they were in his situation. He may also be responsive to a suggestion that he ask others what they would do.

What is rule-bound thinking?

AD children think highly of rules. They believe rules should be followed at all times and by all people. When playing games, they are insistent that others follow the rules and they become furious when other children break or change the rules. He can't let it go and just get back to playing. When his peers break minor school rules, he is the first and often only one to tattle. Unlike his peers who learned as early as kindergarten that you quickly become disliked if you tattle too much, AD children become the classroom and playground police.

While the AD child expects others to achieve perfection in following rules, he is unable to achieve this high standard himself. AD children and teens are usually not intentional rule breakers. However, their inability to tolerate and manage their frustration results in frequent rule infractions in the form of tantrums, outbursts, and defiance.

The good news about rule-bound thinking is that the AD child is less likely to engage in blatant breaking of rules such as stealing and lying when young. When he reaches adolescence he is less likely to engage in smoking, drinking, truancy, and delinquency.

How can I help my child with rule-bound thinking?

Expect your AD child to have difficulty with rule-bound thinking far longer than his peers. While his classmates have learned to tolerate small rule breaking for the sake of keeping a game going or maintaining a friendship, the AD child is very slow to understand this. He applies the concept of rules rigidly with no room for variation.

It may seem odd to set a goal to try to help him accept that sometimes rule breaking is okay, but the reality is that minor infractions happen. You certainly should not encourage him to break rules, but he will get along better with others if he can learn to tolerate it when they break a rule. Expect him to struggle with knowing which rules are "okay" to break and which ones are important to tell an adult when broken. Encourage him to ask for guidance on this. If you see that he has continuing difficulty with determining the difference between acceptable and unacceptable rule infractions, you can make him a list with one column of broken rules to tell an adult and the other column with broken rules he can ignore.

What is truth-bound thinking?

AD children are likely to be honest to the point of cruelty. They do not understand that it is socially inappropriate to say whatever comes to mind. Even when told not to say things that would hurt someone's feelings, the AD child cannot understand what is wrong with telling the truth. They cannot stand in someone else's shoes and understand what it feels like to be told that they are fat or that their hair looks weird. When corrected and told not to say such a thing, the AD child is bewildered and responds, "But it is true."

This may sound like a description of the typical three- or four-year-old child who passes through a stage of saying aloud whatever he sees without regard for the impact it has on others. With coaching, however, most children quickly learn to keep their observations of people's faults to themselves or to at least say it quietly to their parent. The AD child, however, does not understand how something that is true could hurt someone.

How can I help my child with truth-bound thinking?

Understanding that your child is not saying hurtful things in order to be mean can make it easier for you to take the time needed to teach him that the truth must not always be spoken aloud. Expect that you will have to teach him this lesson again and again for several years. Because he does not understand what the insulted person feels like, he will have a very hard time grasping what it is that he is not supposed to say. When he finally grasps the concept that telling people they are ugly is hurtful, he will not be able to generalize this to also know that he should not tell people that their teeth or hair are ugly. Because AD children think very literally and do not apply what they learn to other situations, you can expect them to continue in truth-bound thinking for many years.

If you find that your child is not responding to your verbal teachings, you may find it helpful to make a list of comments that are not okay to say to others. As you hear him make inappropriate comments to others, you can add them to the list that you review with him weekly.

What is perfectionistic thinking?

Perfectionism is intolerance for less-than-perfect performance. Many AD children strive for perfection and become intensely frustrated when they fail to achieve it. This is most often seen during classwork and homework where the AD child may erase his paper over and over, sometimes to the point of tearing it, in his quest to write a word perfectly. His inability to get it "just right" stops him from being able to move on and get his work done.

Perfectionism also appears in the AD child's play. He is far more interested in organizing his special interest collection or telling his playmate all the rules he has created, and leaves little time to actually play. He can't shift gears and start to play even though his playmate may threaten to find someone else to play with.

Most very young children will have several episodes of frustration when they cannot perform a task perfectly. With coaching from their parents, they quickly learn to accept that mistakes are part of life. The AD child, however, has repeated instances of being unable to cope with imperfection in himself and others. Crying, yelling, throwing objects, and quitting the task altogether are common outcomes of perfectionism.

How can I help my child with perfectionist thinking?

You probably are already using good techniques to encourage your child to learn to accept that mistakes are okay and that everyone makes them. When you see him make a mistake, telling him in a gentle voice, "That's okay," "Just keep going," or "Don't worry about that" can help plant thoughts in his mind that he will eventually come to have on his own.

It is very important for you to learn to read your child's frustration level in order to choose the best technique. Very mild frustration in your child's perfectionism calls for a very mild technique on your part. As she becomes increasingly upset, your techniques will increase in intensity, such as in the list below:

- Set the tone at the beginning that mistakes are fine and not to worry about them.
- Interrupt her perfectionist thought pattern by asking if she would like to move on.

- Encourage her to evaluate her mistake by asking what it has to look like before she is happy.
- Encourage her to take a five-minute break and do something fun.
- Create a brief distraction you are certain she will respond to (e.g., let the dog in for her to pet, give her a favorite treat to eat).
- Ask what you can do to help her.
- Ask if she would like you to take it from her so she can stop thinking about it and do her other work instead.
- Give an empathic warning that if she can't stop and move on, you will take it from her so she can stop being so upset and that you will let her come back to it later.
- Take the work from her and direct her to take a break.

What is catastrophic thinking?

Catastrophic thinking refers to viewing upsetting situations as atrocious. What appears to the outside observer to be a trivial problem is viewed as a horrendous, insurmountable problem to the AD child. Because they see things in only shades of black and white, they cannot judge the severity of a problem. Things are either good or really bad—with nothing in between. When something goes wrong, the AD child often views it as devastating.

AD children engage in a lot of catastrophic thinking. Not only do they react to truly upsetting situations with intense distress, they have the same reaction to minor irritations that most children would not even notice. They catastrophize how bad things are and hold the belief that it will forever be awful. From this thought pattern comes intense emotions of anger, frustration, and sadness.

We expect toddlers to have intense reactions when things upset them because they cannot yet put the event into a bigger perspective. They also cannot think about the near future and understand that there is probably a quick solution to the problem. AD children have this same type of thinking pattern. Events are blown out of proportion, and they get stuck in this catastrophic thinking.

How can I help my child with catastrophic thinking?

Catastrophic thinking will be easy for you to recognize in your child. When you are stunned at how upset he is over a trivial event, you can be sure he is having catastrophic thoughts. As with many of the thinking errors of AD, logic and reasoning do not seem to help him calm down. Telling him, "It is not that bad" only works to make him more intent on showing you just how horrible it really is.

Regardless of how minor a situation seems to you, realize that for your child it is a big deal. Rather than persuading him it is not "that bad," encourage him to express his thoughts and feelings: "I see you are upset that Sean looked at your toy. What did you want to have happen?" Then provide empathy and ask him what can be done now: "I know it disappointing to have your surprise ruined. What can we do now?" Don't be surprised if he tells you that "nothing!" can be done. He won't like your suggestion, but at least you are planting seeds for him to learn how to soothe himself and put the upset in perspective. Then you will have to give him room to have his upset and recover in his own time.

What is rigid thinking?

Rigid thinking occurs when individuals become stuck on one viewpoint and cannot think about things in a different way. This is the rigid thinking characteristic of AD children and teens. It shows up in all arenas of life. In play, they cannot be flexible and cooperative with their peers because they have their mind set on how it should be and have no room for alternatives. In school and homework, they are rigid in how they approach the work and are not open to suggestions from parents and teachers; they therefore have trouble completing assignments. In conflicts with others, they are closed off to considering their contribution to the disagreement; therefore, they cannot repair relationships.

It is not difficult to see how rigid thinking interferes in daily life and relationships. The AD child sees the world his way only and believes that everyone else is wrong.

Failure to consider alternative viewpoints and different ways of solving a problem or approaching a task results in the AD child making the same mistakes over and over and over. He cannot benefit from experience because he is not open to ideas different than his own.

How can I help my child with rigid thinking?

The first part of helping your child with rigid thinking is to work on your own frustration level. Understanding that her thought patterns are not intentional stubbornness but a true inability to consider different perspectives can help give you the patience you need. Imagine if you were on one side of a solid door and she were on the other side and you insist she comment on your new haircut. She tells you she can't see it because of the door. You keep insisting that she comment on your haircut. Unless the door opens, she will never be able to see your haircut. On a daily basis, AD children and teens cannot see what is on the other side of the door. Furthermore, they don't even know there is a door that they could open to see what's on the other side.

Over the years, you will have to work at prompting your child to give consideration to different ideas. Always acknowledge your child's viewpoint: "I can see why you would think that," before proposing an alternative: "Here's another way to think about it." Don't insist that you are right and he is wrong. Instead, use language like, "What would you say to . . . ?" Think of it in terms of the old phrase "You can lead a horse to water but you cannot make him drink."

What is perseverative thinking?

Perseverative thinking is when someone gets an idea in their head and just can't get it out. The AD child has perseverative thoughts almost daily. Some parents have used the terms obsessive or compulsive to describe their child's perseverative thinking. However, in true obsessive-compulsive disorder, the perseverative thoughts are unwanted and distressing. In AD, they are usually pleasant and focused on the child's special interest. His repetitive thoughts about his special interest drive him to talk about it again and again and again.

AD children also demonstrate perseverative thinking in school, where they ask endless questions about a specific topic. The AD child may become excited to hear a lesson on the English pilgrims that sailed to America. If he becomes interested in the English ships, he will ask questions about the ships, each one getting more detailed and off the topic of English explorers. The topic of ships gets stuck in his head and he can't stop thinking about it. His teachers and classmates are annoyed, and he has to be directed to stop asking questions about ships. When he gets home, he will talk about ships and ask question after question after question. When you change the topic, he brings it back to ships.

How can I help my child with perseverative thinking?

There is no real answer as where to draw the line in stopping your child from perseverating on a topic and allowing him the freedom to think and be inquisitive.

You certainly want to encourage your child to learn, ask questions, and become excited about different topics. However, you probably don't want to talk about airplane engines for three hours, and neither does the rest of the world. There are also many instances where perseverative thinking can interfere and distract him and he will need you to help interrupt the thought pattern.

In the classroom, his teacher can stop perseverative questioning by telling him, "One more question and then we will get back to the lesson." Parents, relatives, and other adults can use the same technique. If your child persists beyond one more question, he can be reminded, "We are not talking about clocks anymore; now we are talking about what movie we will see tonight." Or he can be told when it is okay to revisit the topic of clocks: "We are not talking about clocks anymore, but tonight at bedtime we can talk about them again."

What is generalization?

Generalization is a term used to refer to learning in one setting that is automatically carried over to other settings. If your child learns that he must raise his hand in school, he will likely raise his hand in Sunday school even without being specifically taught to do so. He has generalized learning from one situation to a similar situation.

Most children generalize learning easily. If you teach them it is wrong to steal candy from a store, they automatically figure out that it is also wrong to steal cookies. AD children, however, are very poor at generalizing and do not learn from experience. Being disciplined for hitting a peer on the playground does not result in learning that he also should not hit a peer on the bus.

Failure to generalize is one of the difficulties in treatment for AD children. What they learn in therapy often does not generalize. While they may become very skilled at using their communication skills in family therapy, when they get home, it is as if they never even heard of communication skills. Some parents have reported that their AD children have told them, "Those skills are only for when we are in therapy, not for when we are home!"

How can I help my child with generalization?

Fortunately, with your help, your child will learn to generalize. Parents are the key to teaching children how to apply their skills in other settings. Being actively involved in learning the same skills as your child and practicing them with him will lead to success. He can go to the most prestigious school and have therapy with the most renowned psychologist, but if you do not use the skills in your daily life, do not expect him to.

Some therapists will give you a workbook or handouts to help you make new skills part of your family's daily life. Scheduling private periodic sessions with your child's therapist to learn what he is being taught and how you can reinforce the lessons at home is also a good idea.

When you discuss a rule, behavior, or problem with your child, ask, "Where do we have to do this rule?" Join your child as she is reciting the list of places. Written or picture lists can be helpful reminders for particular problems your child has trouble generalizing. You can pleasantly reflect on a previous problem situation and remind him that the current situation is just like the other one.

Chapter 6

EMOTIONAL INTELLIGENCE

- What is emotional intelligence?
- Why is emotional intelligence important?
- What are the emotional problems of children and teens with Asperger's Disorder?
- Do children and teens with Asperger's Disorder recognize emotions in others?
- Do children and teens with Asperger's Disorder experience empathy?
- Can children and teens with Asperger's Disorder learn empathy?
- Are children and teens with Asperger's Disorder critical of others?
- How can I teach my child or teen empathy?
- How can I teach my child or teen advanced empathy?
- Should I have my child apologize when he lacks empathy?
- How do children and teens with Asperger's Disorder express feelings?
- What causes children and teens with Asperger's Disorder to have intense emotions?
- Can children and teens with Asperger's Disorder be taught feelings?
- How do I help my child learn about emotions?
- What is emotional regulation?
- How can I help my child with emotional regulation?
- How can playing help my child with emotions?
- How can charades help my child with emotions?
- How can collages help my child with emotions?
- How can journaling help my child with feelings?
- How can movies help my child with emotions?

What is emotional intelligence?

Completely independent from IQ, emotional intelligence, abbreviated as EQ, refers to how attuned someone is to feelings. We are born with an emotional intelligence that allows us to feel, use, communicate, recognize, remember, learn from, manage, and understand emotions. Those with high emotional intelligence are attuned both to the feelings of others as well as their own. They understand people's moods, motivations, and desires.

Emotional intelligence allows us to recognize, identify, and express feelings. We do this through reading facial expressions, body language, and tone of voice, and considering these in the context in which they are expressed. We are able to correctly label our own feelings as well as others' feelings and talk about, express, and manage them appropriately.

Emotional intelligence also allows us to use feelings in problem solving and decision making. It allows us to see the connection between thoughts, feelings, and behavior. With higher levels of emotional intelligence, we can understand how emotions change from one to other and how we can experience more than one feeling at a time, and sometimes have simultaneous feelings that are contradictory.

Why is emotional intelligence important?

Many psychologists believe that emotional intelligence is exceedingly more important than academic intelligence. Being book smart only carries one so far in life and does little for personal relationships. Those with the highest skills in emotional intelligence have happy lives, successful marriages, close friendships, and high self-esteem. They intuitively use emotional intelligence to draw others to them and make others feel good being in their company. They make good leaders who can resolve conflicts, manage people, and motivate others.

Psychologists estimate that 80–90 percent of our communication is nonverbal. Through nonverbal social cues of body language, tone of voice, facial expression, and display of emotions, we let others know who we are, what we think, how we feel, what we believe, and what we want. If someone is blind to this type of communication and can only understand spoken words, it is easy to understand why he does not understand people. He cannot form even a basic sense of connection to others in childhood. As we get older, communication becomes more complex in meaning, but at the same time more subtle in expression, leaving those with poor emotional intelligence even more confused and lost in their attempts to relate to others.

What are the emotional problems of children and teens with Asperger's Disorder?

Children and teens with AD have limited interest in emotions—both their own and those of others. They do not try to understand how others feel, nor do they change their words or behavior in reaction to others. Their emotional blindness renders them incapable of recognizing a peer's irritation, boredom, or impatience. Even when emotions are openly expressed by others, children with AD do not respond with empathy. They lack both an intellectual and emotional understanding of how others feel and often respond in inappropriate and insensitive ways. Their failure to notice emotions and modify their words and actions is not rude or callous; they simply do not see or feel emotions they way others do.

Some of the difficulties AD children and teens have with emotions include:

- Being aware that others have feelings
- Recognizing when someone has a feeling
- Reading others' facial expressions
- Correctly identifying a person's feeling
- Giving an appropriate response to the feelings
- Recognizing when they are having a feeling
- Correctly labeling their own feeling
- Using facial expressions to convey their feeling
- Expressing their feeling with appropriate intensity

Do children and teens with Asperger's Disorder recognize emotions in others?

Children and teens with AD are unable to recognize that someone is experiencing an emotion. When people display their feelings, people with AD literally do not notice it. The primary reason seems to be that they lack an understanding that all people have feelings. While we do not consciously think about it, most of us operate in the social world with the understanding that all humans are emotional beings and that we need to be careful about what we say and do in order to try to avoid hurting others. If you had AD, you would not have this understanding and would give the same weight to other people's feelings as you would to the feelings of furniture.

Another contributor to this symptom is the finding that children with AD do not look into the eyes of people they are listening to. Most people make mutual eye contact during a conversation. AD children and teens, however, look at other parts of the face or the body or even objects in the environment. They miss out on the easy clues that eye contact can provide about what another person is feeling.

Do children and teens with Asperger's Disorder experience empathy?

Children and teens with AD are often accused of being selfish and insensitive to the feelings of others. Their lack of responsiveness, failure to ask the other person about their feelings, and changing the topic to themselves appears to lack sensitivity. While this type of behavior is insensitive, the intention is not. They simply do not register and interpret people's emotions. They do not see the emotions, hear them, or feel them like most people do. Nor do they understand how another person feels. The AD child is really clueless as to how others feel. The insensitive things they say and do is a result of not attributing emotions to other people. Odd as it seems, even though they certainly know what it feels like to have someone hurt their feelings, they do not grasp that others have the same emotional experiences that they do. They understand the emotions of people about as well as we understand the emotional life of an aardvark.

Can children and teens with Asperger's Disorder learn empathy?

Most children do not need to be taught empathy. Even infants physically close to one another display empathy by crying when the other one does. Babies will crawl over to gently pat another crying baby or bring them an object to soothe them. Toddlers can identify how others are feeling. In contrast, AD children do not display these behaviors because they lack empathy. Think of them as emotionally blind, not seeing emotions in others.

Empathy *can* be taught. It is a long-term process that may never be fully complete. Most adults with AD say that while they learned that in order to get along in the world they had to pay attention to how other people feel, they still do not truly understand it emotionally.

They have learned to act as if they have empathy, even if they do not feel it. Using a mental checklist, they have to ask themselves, "What is the person feeling?" and "What is the appropriate response I should make for this particular feeling?"

Are children and teens with Asperger's Disorder critical of others?

By age five or six, children learn to keep their negative observations about others to themselves. They no longer blurt out the embarrassing comments common to three- and four-year-olds who do not yet understand that people feel bad if tell them, "You are fat."

AD children, however, seem to take pride in pointing out the faults of others, and they have no hesitancy doing so in front of others. Not only do they point out the faults of their peers they have no discomfort in pointing out the faults of adults and authority figures. Their feedback to adults and peers alike is filled with sentences starting with, "You should..." They do not gently give a helpful suggestion, but a statement that clearly lets you know that what you are doing is inadequate and you obviously need to be told what to do instead. As a group leader, I have had AD children tell me how I should run the group, what words I should use for my lesson plans, and how I should give a time-out. They are blind to how their authoritative and confident manner gives off a sense of arrogance and insensitivity.

How can I teach my child or teen empathy?

You are sure to have plenty of opportunities to teach lessons of empathy to your child.

When you observe him saying or doing something that seems mean or insensitive, try to recall that this is most likely due his inability to understand how the other person feels. Instead of punishment, you can use the moment to teach empathy. The calmer and more understanding you can be, the more willing your child will be to listen to you. Tell him what you saw him do or what your heard him say and ask him, "How do you think Leon feels about you calling him an idiot?" Don't be surprised if he does not answer you, as he may not know how Leon feels, in which case you will tell him that Leon feels mad and sad. If he has learned from your teaching that kids feel bad when they are called names, he may tell you, "Leon feels bad." This shows the beginning stages of empathy. Don't assume, however, that just because he can label the feeling, that he has an emotional understanding of how the other person feels. He will have to spend several years simply learning how other people feel before he begins to have some emotional sense.

How can I teach my child or teen advanced empathy?

Once your child has a consistent understanding that his words and actions can make someone feel bad, you can add more advanced lessons. Teach him why Leon feels bad when he is called an idiot. Initially you will have to tell him, "Leon feels bad when you call him an idiot because it makes him think you don't like him, that you think he is stupid, and that you don't want to be his friend." Asking him if this is how he meant to make Leon feel should result in a "no." If by chance he says yes, you know that he is not ready yet to talk about it and that he and Leon need to be separated for a while. Revisit the issue later when he is calm.

The goal is for your child to eventually be able to state the effect his words have on others without having to rely on you to tell him. Expect this to take years, not months. Be sure to help him understand how his words and actions can also make others feel good.

Should I have my child apologize when he lacks empathy?

Everyone should apologize when they hurt someone. The AD child is sure to hurt the feelings of more people than the average person over his lifetime. One of the best relationship tools you can give him is the skill of making a good apology. A well thought out and sincere apology can go a very long way in repairing a relationship. Your child will be able to find more tolerance and forgiveness for his repeated social offenses if he readily makes apologies.

A good start is to simply help your child to say he is sorry. The more he learns about empathy the easier it will be for him to add more to his apology. Expect this to be a long-term project that you will work on throughout his childhood and adolescence.

A meaningful apology includes the following elements:

• You are sorry: "I am sorry, Grandma."
• You admit you did something wrong: "I should not have said I hate you."
• You explain what you did: "I just got so mad that I forgot to control my words."
• You understand that they were hurt: "I know I hurt your feelings."
• You understand how they feel: "I know you probably feel mad at me."
• You did not intend to hurt them: "I did not want to hurt your feelings."
• You want to fix the hurt: "Can I do something to stop your hurt feelings?"
• You want to keep the relationship: "I love you and appreciate all you do for me."
• You want to be forgiven: "I hope you can forgive me."

How do children and teens with Asperger's Disorder express feelings?

The way in which children and teens with AD express their feelings can be unpredictable. At times they seem emotionally flat, as if they have no emotion whatsoever. This leaves other people feeling uncomfortable. It is awkward to interact with someone who shows no feelings. Our culture is so sociable and emotionally interactive that when people encounter an emotionally flat AD child or teen they perceive them as weird, mechanical, or robotic.

At other times, the emotions of AD children are dramatic and out of proportion to the situation. Their emotional displays are extremely immature and more consistent with those of a pre-schooler. Even AD teenagers can react with the emotional maturity of a first-grader. While these outbursts might seem to have no apparent cause, they are usually the result of frustration from the child feeling trapped in a problem he cannot solve or a situation he cannot control or escape from. Recall his thinking problems from chapter 5. This should make it easier to understand why AD children become emotionally overwhelmed.

There seems to be little range between flat emotions and intense reactions. This can feel like an emotional roller coaster where you are probably inclined to prefer your child's unemotional state.

What causes children and teens with Asperger's Disorder to have intense emotions?

There are some general patterns that children and teens with AD have when they are most likely to react with emotional intensity:

- When they feel someone is invading their physical space
- When things are unpredictable
- When they are in new situations
- When they are not in control of the situation
- When they cannot predict what will happen next

Certainly, these situations cannot always be prevented. However, as often as you can set things up so these types of events do not happen, the fewer episodes your child will have. Having a highly organized household and daily routine will decrease outbursts. Using charts, calendars, and lists helps create predictability. Warning your child in advance of upcoming changes gives her time to emotionally accept the disruption in her routine.

Your child likely has other situations that cause him upset. It helps to keep a diary of the day's events and note your child's behavior and mood. Over time, when you reread your diary, you are likely to find patterns of situations that result in upset. As much as you can alter those situations to prevent the upset, the less instances of distress your child will have.

Can children and teens with Asperger's Disorder be taught feelings?

Understanding emotions and how they impact social relationships escapes those with AD. Most children learn about feelings through experiencing them. AD children, however, need to have formal instruction in feelings. One goal is to teach them about their own feelings while another is to teach them about other people's feelings. You can expect greater success in teaching them about their own feelings than those of others. This is because they experience their own feelings and they therefore can learn to identify and express them appropriately. Their poor empathy makes it more difficult for those with AD to learn about the feelings of others.

Learning about their own feelings can be done through a variety of children's storybooks, workbooks, and group or individual therapy. Lessons are direct teaching of what the various feelings are, what they look like on people's faces, how they feel in our body, and how to express them appropriately.

While it seems logical that from learning about their own feelings children with AD would be able to generalize this to other people, this simply does not happen. They must have additional instruction about how other people feel and how to respond appropriately.

How do I help my child learn about emotions?

The first skill to teach your child is the many emotions we all experience. Don't assume that just because your child shows some emotions he has a good understanding of them. A simple and fun tool for learning feelings is to hang a poster in her room of feeling faces. Most children and teens enjoy finding their feelings on the poster. You will know if your child is gaining understanding about feelings when she begins to use feeling words in her talk. When you hear her say, "I was so mad today!" or "Daddy, that hurts my feelings," you know she is attending to her emotions and seeking to share them with you.

The next phase is to teach a more advanced lesson in feelings by introducing the range of intensity of various feelings. When we are angry we can be irritated, annoyed, mad, furious, or rageful, depending on how intense we feel. When we are happy we can be pleased, content, excited, thrilled, or ecstatic. Learning these labels can help children learn to assess the depth or intensity of their feelings, which can help guide their choices in how they will display and control their feelings.

FEELINGS

Positive	Negative
Happy	Sad
Determined	Mad
Joyful	Scared
Pleased	Jealous
Comfortable	Uncomfortable
Loved	Lonely
Appreciated	Depressed
Accepted	Disgusted
Peaceful	Nervous
Relieved	Frustrated
Inspired	Guilty
Confident	Resentful
Glad	Embarrassed
Encouraged	Discouraged
Proud	Ashamed
Excited	Bored
Optimistic	Afraid
Satisfied	Confused
Relaxed	Worried
Amused	Worthless
Interested	Fed-up
Capable	Dissatisfied
Worthy	Hurt
Concerned	Shocked
Curious	Trapped
Eager	Humiliated

FEELINGS *continued*

Positive	Negative
Optimistic	Terrified
Courageous	Infuriated
Hopeful	Annoyed
Brave	Helpless
Cheerful	Lethargic
Delighted	Regretful
Calm	Shy
Good	Unsure
Eager	Hesitant
Grateful	Suspicious
Friendly	Self-conscious
Playful	Disappointed

What is emotional regulation?

Emotional regulation is the ability to control one's emotional expression. Early signs of AD as well as many other childhood psychological disorders begin with troubles with emotional regulation. Until their child is diagnosed with AD, many parents do not recognize their child's emotional flatness as a problem. Instead it is their child's intense emotional reactions that often call attention to the disorder.

Being able to regulate or manage our emotions is necessary to function in every setting. Every child faces multiple situations each day that have the potential for upset. Through early teaching from their parents, nondisordered children learn how to regulate their feelings. They learn to not react to trivial upsets and just let them go. They learn that when they are angry, they must control their temper. They learn how to seek support from others or how to soothe themselves when they are sad. They also learn how to have their behavior consistent with the intensity of their feeling. Like a pressure valve on a hose, emotional regulation allows us to control how much emotion we let out. AD children and teens do not have this type of pressure valve. Instead they seem to simply have an on/off switch.

How can I help my child with emotional regulation?

Teaching your child to regulate his emotions can be done with a variety of methods. Because anger is the most difficult feeling for most people to manage, and particularly for those with AD, this will likely be the feeling you will focus on the most. You can teach your child skills of:

- Deep breathing: slow, deep breaths to calm down the body and interrupt behavior
- Muscle relaxation: squeezing and releasing muscles to decrease physical tension
- Visualization: imagining a happy scene to replace angry thoughts
- Thought stopping: imagining a stop sign to stop the angry thoughts
- Thought replacement: focusing on a more pleasant or reasonable thought
- Thought disputing: thinking about why your angry thoughts are inaccurate
- Count down: counting backwards from twenty to interrupt angry thoughts
- Distraction: engaging in a distracting and pleasant activity
- Journaling: drawing or writing about the angry feelings
- Talking: telling someone about the angry feelings
- Physical activity: releasing the anger by running, throwing a ball, etc.

These skills are not just for children and teens. The better job you do regulating your emotions, the easier it will be for your child to regulate his. If you use the vocabulary of emotional regulation, you help instill it in your child's mind. You can guide him in using the variety of skills when you see him struggling to calm himself down.

There are many fun activity workbooks for children about anger management that you and your child can do together. You can find a list of these workbooks in the Appendix.

How can playing help my child with emotions?

Most of us learn emotions from interacting with others and observing how people express their feelings with their faces, bodies, and words. For the AD child, the language of feelings is foreign to them and they do not easily learn what comes smoothly to others. AD children need to be taught emotions in a very direct way, much like you would teach them any new skill. Direct instruction can be boring, tedious, tiresome, and an unnatural way for AD children to gain experience with emotions. Instead, many fun activities can be used with your child to help him learn emotions. The idea is to slip in teaching opportunities in the form of play without your child necessarily knowing that the purpose is to teach. Art projects and various games are ways to have fun with your child while teaching him valuable lessons. There are board games and storybooks specifically designed to teach feelings. Playing house, dolls, or school can provide plenty of opportunity to focus on feelings.

You do not want to say, "Now we are going to learn about feelings." Instead suggest a game of charades, making a collage, finger painting, or other activities suggested in this chapter.

How can charades help my child with emotions?

Most adults and children are familiar with the game of charades. One person acts out a behavior, word, phrase, thought, or feeling, and the other players have to guess what it is. AD children can be good at guessing behaviors or words but are quite poor at guessing feelings. Playing charades where the focus is on acting out feelings gives the AD child a fun way to learn how to read the emotions of others.

Your child may not want to act out feelings and probably will prefer to act out something related to his favorite interest. This is fine because you can be the one to act out emotions and have him guess what feeling you have. Charades involve hand signals at the beginning so the players know what category to guess in. You can create a feelings signal by making a big smile and tracing your finger over your mouth. Your child has to guess what behavior and/or situation you are doing and what feeling you are having about the behavior. Look to your child's feelings poster to be sure to vary the feelings you act out.

How can collages help my child with emotions?

Many children love to make collages where they take pictures from magazines and glue them on poster board. Collages are a fun way for children to learn to read the emotions of other people. Don't worry if your child is resistant to finding pictures of feelings or people. Let him choose whatever he likes and you can choose the feelings. On some occasions you can set it up so that he chooses his collage topic and you choose yours, which of course will be feelings. Set a timer and when it goes off after five minutes, you have to switch seats and work on the other person's collage for the next five minutes. This not only helps your child gain the experience of looking at people's faces and reading their emotions, but provides him with an opportunity to gain another person's perspective when he changes seats with you and has to now work on your project.

As your child gains experience with feelings, you can switch from feelings in general to a specific feeling so that your collage will have only pictures of people have one particular feeling. This gives your child the chance to pay more attention to the various emotional expressions of people's faces.

How can journaling help my child with feelings?

Journaling is one way to help your child express his feelings and write about what happened during his day. You will increase the chances of your child becoming interested in journaling if you yourself journal. You can set aside a five- to fifteen-minute period each day when you and your child sit together and do your journaling. You each write about your day. When you are finished, you each can share what you wrote if you want to. If your child wants to keep it private, allow him to do so. If he wants to share it with you, be sure to listen and keep your comments brief and supportive. This is not a time to teach or lecture. You want him to feel safe sharing his thoughts and feelings. If he writes in his journal that two boys knocked over his sandcastle and laughed at him so he chased then and hit them as hard as he could, resist the temptation to turn this into a talk about how we don't hit and what he should have done differently. Instead give him empathy and support with a comment to the effect of, "That sounds like a rough situation and I'm guessing it made you pretty mad." You are providing empathy and inviting him to talk about his feelings. He may talk or may only say yes. If he only says yes, that he was mad and that's it, ask him if he would like to talk about it anymore. If he says no, respect that and ask if there is anything you can do, and let him know if he wants to talk about it another time you are there to listen.

To help model what to put in a journal, what feelings to write about, and how to share your day and emotions with others, be sure to read your entry to your child even if he wants to keep his private. Of course you will put entries that are appropriate for a child to hear and not burden him with your troubles or emotions. Try to include things that caused emotions so that he hears that events cause feelings, what feelings you had, and how you handled them. On occasion, you can decline to share and say you want to keep today's entry private to model this for him. Write about both positive and negative feelings and positive and negative outcomes.

SAMPLE JOURNAL ENTRY

Positive Emotions
Today when I read my email, I was *excited* when I had an email from Aunt Teri. I got a big *smile* on my face when I read that she got a new puppy. When I read that the puppy chewed up her new shoes, I felt *sorry* for her because I know those are her favorite. When I was done reading the email, I called Aunt Teri to thank her for sharing the news about the puppy and tell her I was sorry to hear about her shoes. I got even *more excited* when she said she would bring the puppy to see us in two weeks. Because of this good news, I have been *happy* all day.

This entry shows the cause and effect of positive feelings. It also shows empathy for the aunt who lost her shoes.

Negative Emotions

Today I was very *happy* because I was driving to meet Grandma for lunch, but then I got a flat tire. I was *scared* when I felt the tire go flat and *nervous* until I could pull the car to the side of the road. Luckily, I had my phone with me and I could call the auto club to fix it for me. I was *mad* because this is the second flat tire I had this summer. I was *upset* that I was going to be late for lunch with Grandma, and I was *worried* that she would be *impatient* with me for being late. I called her to apologize and she made me *feel better* when she told me *not to worry* about being late; she just wanted me safe, and she would wait for me. The tire man was *very nice* and I felt *very relieved* once he changed the tire. Grandma was nice too when I finally got there, and we had a good lunch.

This entry shows a variety of emotions and shows how feelings can change quickly. It also shows how we can guess how someone else is going to feel.

How can movies help my child with emotions?

Movies are filled with a wide variety of feelings and are a great tool to teach emotions. As with the other activities in this chapter, watching movies at home with your child must be a fun event, not a structured lesson for learning. Most children are talkative and inquisitive during movies, often asking, "Why did he do that?" "What's he going to do next?" or "Why is he mad?" While this can be irritating if you are also trying to enjoy the movie, choose specific times when you can make the teaching of emotions your goal and you can answer all his questions.

Animated children's movies can be an even better tool for teaching emotions than those with actors. Animation is usually done with dramatic facial expressions that are easy to read. The character's faces are also left on the screen for a longer period of time, giving the child time to look at the face and think about what the character is feeling. The dialogue in children's animation is also often very simple, and the other characters in the movie usually verbalize what the other characters are feeling, making it easier for children to follow the story. Disney and Pixar animations do an excellent job of showing emotions and teaching about friendship, loyalty, and empathy. Characters usually have many feelings that they openly share with another character. They also usually face a challenge they must overcome, but only if they seek the help of others.

You can occasionally make a comment about the character's feelings to help aid your child in reading emotions. Comments such as, "Oh, he looks so sad!" or "Oh my, is he ever angry!" help label feelings and at the same time demonstrates your empathy for the characters.

Oftentimes children are so excited by a movie that they talk about it for days afterwards. This is a great opportunity to keep the feeling and the emotional message of the movie on your child's mind. However, if he does not talk about it spontaneously, you can try a few times to start a conversation about it, but if he does not respond, let it go so he does not learn that each time he watches a movie with you it becomes a lesson.

Chapter 7

SPECIAL INTERESTS, ROUTINES, AND PLAY

- What are the interest patterns of children and teens with Asperger's Disorder?
- Why do children with Asperger's Disorder have intense interests?
- How do I tell if my child's interest is a problem?
- What should I do about my child's intense interest?
- Does my child's special interest provide any benefits?
- Can a club be of help to my child?
- Should I participate in my child's special interest?
- Will my child's special interests cause problems at school?
- How can my child's teacher help with special interests?
- Will my child outgrow his special interest?
- Are children and teens with Asperger's Disorder insistent on routine and sameness?
- Why is routine and sameness important for children and teens with Asperger's Disorder?
- How should I respond to my child's insistence on routine and sameness?
- How can I increase my child's flexibility?
- How can my child's teacher help with insistence on routine and sameness?
- How can my child's teacher help with flexibility?
- How does the insistence on routine and sameness affect my child's play?
- How do special interests affect my child's play?
- What are normal play patterns?
- What should I look for in my child's play?
- What are the play difficulties of children and teens with Asperger's Disorder?
- Why is play so important?
- How do I know if my child has play problems?
- Should I encourage my child to play with others?
- How can I help my child improve play skills?
- How can playdates help improve my child's social skills?
- What kind of activities can help my child's play skills?
- What type of peer should my child play with?

What are the interest patterns of children and teens with Asperger's Disorder?

One of the hallmark symptoms of AD is the intense preoccupation with a specific interest. AD children become almost obsessed with a particular toy, topic, or object, and the rest of the world holds little interest for them. Often their interest involves collecting items and arranging them over and over in a rather meaningless way. They may develop repetitive routines with their items that have little meaning and are performed in a rote manner.

The interests are usually done alone, with little or no interest in sharing the pleasure with others. Sharing with others is not a mutual exchange of fun ideas and knowledge, but an endless drone of knowledge. The interest is one they found on their own and not selected by parents, teachers, or friends. They do not care if others are not interested; they do not succumb to peer pressure to drop their interest and pursue what the other kids are into. Their interest may be a common interest, such as dinosaurs or World War II battleships, or it may be very unique, such as locks or bottle tops. Some parents have used the word fanatical to describe their child's intense and restricted interest.

Why do children and teens with Asperger's Disorder have intense interests?

The interest dominates their time, thoughts, and conversations. In a world where they are usually the odd man out, their interest provides an opportunity to shine as the most knowledgeable one in the group. This showing off of advanced and detailed knowledge, however, is not often seen as a desirable trait, and peers and adults alike may find themselves seeking polite ways to get out of the situation.

Giving a monologue on the topic may also provide a sense of relaxation for the AD child. The monotone, nonstop talking about information can be almost meditative, as the AD child quickly gets himself into a state where he can go on and on and on.

Special interests may also be pursued as the most predictable source of pleasure for the AD child. People are not very enticing to AD children, but objects are. Their specific interest can be the only thing in life they can consistently find pleasure in.

When other activities, toys, objects, or topics are suggested or introduced, the AD child is either unresponsive or resistant. He likes what he likes and has no need for variety.

How do I tell if my child's interest is a problem?

It is common for most children and teens to have one or two things they are very interested in. Your child may be interested in *Star Wars* and want to decorate his room in this theme, collect all the figures, wear the pajamas, read the books, watch the movies over and over, collect the cards, and dress as one of the characters for Halloween. Is he an enthusiastic collector or a disordered child? It is hard to know where to draw the line.

On one hand, a special interest that interferes with a child's ability to interact with others is surely a problem. If he can talk about little else, is insistent that his peers play only his special interest, and refuses to do schoolwork unrelated to his special interest, then it has crossed over from an enthusiastic hobby to a problem. On the other hand, if a special interest provides a great source of pleasure, increases knowledge, and enhances self-esteem, it can be hard to actually say it is a problem. Behaviors are usually determined to be a problem if they interfere with functioning. Your child's interest may provide a mixture of problems and pleasure.

What should I do about my child's intense interest?

Presently there is no clear answer as to the best way to handle special interests. Two schools of thought exist. One is to try to decrease the interest, and the second is to allow the interest to improve the child's life.

Professionals who find interests to be problematic view the child's life and world experience as restricted and believe that the child needs to be exposed to other interests. They suggest that the child's favorite interest be limited in time so that he has no choice but to find something else to occupy his time. Purposeful exposure to other interests is suggested in the hope that the child will find other things that he likes. No research yet exists to tell us whether or not this is a good idea.

Another approach is to view the special interest as a unique trait, not as something to be fixed. Many parents report that their AD child is happiest when engaged in his interest. Countless adults have turned their childhood interest into a career or a lifelong hobby and source of pleasure.

The general consensus of professionals is to allow for the special interest while also exposing AD children and teens to other potential interests.

Does my child's special interest provide any benefits?

Like anyone with an interest or hobby, the special interest of your AD child provides pleasure. His level of enjoyment is probably equal to his level of obsession.

Self-esteem is somewhat tied to special interests. Your child is probably very good at his interest. He is likely to be knowledgeable, careful about his collection, and derive a sense of accomplishment. He also can use his special interest as a retreat from the stresses of the day. He can be in complete control of his interest and no one can tell him he is doing it wrong.

The chance to develop friendships may also arise out of your child's special interest. For AD children who do not know how to start conversations or maintain one, or do not know how to keep a friend, a special interest provides a common ground. If your child's special interest is a popular one with his peer group, he is likely to have moments when he fits in. Some studies have found that the level of social skills improves for AD children during the time they are talking and playing with another AD child who shares their same interest. Two AD children that have the same special interest can feel as if they have found their soul mate.

Can a club be of help to my child?

A club that focuses on your child's special interest may be the only place where he feels he truly belongs. If he can find a group of peers who share his passion for his interest, then he finds acceptance and most likely a friend. Don't be concerned if the friendship is focused solely on the interest. If he and his friend are happy with this, then they have each found what they want. This is certainly better than having no friends. If your child has an interest, chances are someone else out there shares his same interest.

Finding a club for your child's interest can be as simple as joining one at school. Your local newspaper, community center, and yellow pages are good sources. Other parents may know of a club. The Internet is a good place to look as well. Stores that sell items related to his special interest usually have other enthusiasts and often have club meetings at their store. If you cannot find a club for your child's interest, you can be the trendsetter and start one. Post flyers at your child's school, temple or church, or at his day care.

Should I participate in my child's special interest?

Setting aside dedicated time to join your child in his special interest is one way to strengthen your relationship. For many adults, some of their fondest memories from childhood are the occasions when their parents spent time playing with them. AD children are no different and crave the same special time with their parents.

A special playdate each week for you and your child to enjoy her interest can serve many purposes. She will feel accepted by you and feel good that you are sharing her interest. By making a special date on the calendar with your child, you help prevent her from relentlessly asking you to play with her or listen to her latest monologue about her interest. Instead you can enthusiastically let her know you see her excitement and you are looking forward to your special playdate when she can tell you all about her latest discovery. This is a pleasant way to prompt her to stop talking about it now and hold her thoughts until your playdate. She then has a time to look forward to and can do a better job of holding it in until then.

Will my child's special interest cause problems at school?

Not all AD children are affected in school by their special interest. They are able to keep their talk and play limited to the playground and at home. Some, however, have difficulty keeping their special interest out of their minds during school. They may attempt to inject their special interest into class discussions regardless of the topic at hand. They monopolize class discussions, ask endless questions of the teacher, and have trouble shifting to a new topic. Resistance to learning other subjects may come in outright refusal, procrastination, or poor effort. Some may lack respect for their teacher's knowledge and seem to have no hesitancy in pointing out the teacher's inaccuracies.

They may try to take over the lesson and attempt to lecture to the teacher and the class about their interest.

Social problems can occur as the result of special interests. Their AD child's advanced vocabulary and factual knowledge about their special interest can give the impression of being a know-it-all. Peers may also find it tiresome to hear about the same topic over and over, and therefore are unlikely to choose the AD child as a playmate.

How can my child's teacher help with special interests?

Teachers who understand that special interests are a symptom of AD will be able to have the patience needed to manage the questions, interruptions, and lectures they are bound to experience.

To help with excessive talk and questions, teachers can:

- Set a specific time, the same time each day, that he can talk about his special interest.
- Interrupt talk about special interests with a reminder of when he can talk about it.
- Prompt the class that each child may ask a designated number of questions.
- Announce that extra questions can be written down to ask during free time.
- Time to talk about, read, or use the Internet to learn about his special interest can be used as reinforcement for completion of other assignments.

Your child's teacher may appreciate your input on ways to help your child incorporate his special interest into his lessons.

Some suggestions teachers can use to help with resistance to doing work unrelated to the special interest include:

- Set the expectation that all assignments, even outside her interest, are to be completed.
- Allow the interest to be incorporated into some assignments (e.g., selecting a book for a book report, choosing a science experiment, writing about the interest on a grammar and punctuation lesson).
- Incorporate the interest into as many lessons as possible (e.g., count the insects, write a story about insects, draw an insect after each spelling word).
- Use his interest to incorporate several subjects at a time. An interest in clocks can include the history of the clock, what was occurring in the world when the clock was invented, how different countries make clocks, which cultures use clocks and which do not, how many more clocks are sold in Japan than the USA.

Will my child outgrow his special interest?

There is no way to predict how long your child will keep his special interest. Some children will change interests over time, passionately pursuing one topic only to later drop it and replace it with another. However, in general it seems that the special interests of AD children persist for years. Their area of focus usually matures as they grow, but the topic may remain the same. Children interested in anime comic books will collect them for years; later they trade them, become interested in reading the collector magazines, start to keep track of the monetary value of each comic book, and later engage in selling and buying comic books to increase the value of their collection. Such a special interest can hold their fascination from elementary through high school years. It is not unusual for a special interest to turn into a career. College or trade school in graphic arts or animation may be the outcome of a childhood interest in comic books. An interest in insects may lead to a degree in biology and career as an entomologist. A child who collects locks may become a locksmith. While not all special interests lead to careers, they do provide a great source of pleasure that many non-AD individuals never experience.

Are children and teens with Asperger's Disorder insistent on routine and sameness?

Many children and teens with AD are insistent on routine and sameness. They want things to go the same every day and react with upset when changes occur. When changes in the daily routine occur, they may have mood changes, behavior problems, and anger outbursts. These may not be displayed at the moment the change happens, making it difficult to see how the change in routine caused the problem.

Their difficulty may show up several hours after the change, seeming to be coming out of nowhere. Changes in routine such as arriving to school late because of traffic, not having his favorite cereal in the cupboard for breakfast, or Dad driving him to school instead of Mom can result in problems. Upset with changes also occur at school. Surprise events such as a fire drill or a substitute teacher can upset a child for the entire day.

Some children with AD are able to express their upset with the change. They may question repeatedly, whine, cry, or refuse to go along with the change. Others, however, give no indication that they are upset and only later do their difficulties coping surface.

Why is routine and sameness important for children and teens with Asperger's Disorder?

Routine helps the AD child move through the world in a predictable way without having to mentally and emotionally face the unexpected.

This is more necessary for the AD child than the average child. Most of us like predictability. We don't like the unexpected. We are creatures of habit who find comfort in the familiar. We go to the same grocery, gym, and post office, and drive the same route to work. Imagine that your grocery was demolished overnight, your gym closed down, and the freeway was closed with no detour signs. Changes in the AD child's daily routine feel like this to him every day. Unpredictable changes for the AD child are like an adult going out to the garage and finding out his car has been replaced by a unicycle.

The AD child's brain is like a computer that can only run one program at a time. Our computers can run the Internet, a word-processing program, and a photo editing program all at the same time. The AD child cannot do this. His computer will crash if the file he is using is interrupted by another file opening unexpectedly.

How should I respond to my child's insistence on routine and sameness?

The good news about the AD child's insistence on sameness is that it can be relatively easy to respond to. The vast majority of people of all ages function better with routine, structure, and predictability in their life. Some AD children and teens just take it to the extreme and have difficulty adjusting to changes.

If your child does have troubles managing her mood and behavior when changes in her daily routine occur, it is best to try to provide her with as much predictability as you can. This means creating a highly structured household where things are physically in order and daily tasks take place in a certain order. Charts, lists, and calendars on the wall help your child to see what will happen each day. Dry-erase boards, bulletin boards with individual cards for each task that you can move around with pins, or calendars you make on your computer will make it easy for you to post the changes without having to recreate the list every time there is a change. Warning her ahead of time of upcoming changes can help prevent upset or minimize it.

How can I increase my child's flexibility?

If your child is rigid and insistent on routine, your goal is not to get rid of this trait, but instead increase his flexibility. No matter how structured and routine you set up your household and your child's life, changes will certainly happen. Because of this, there is no need to purposely create disruptions in the routine in order to expose your child to change. You will be faced with helping your child cope with both predictable and unpredictable changes.

Predictable changes will be easier to help your child adjust to. Upcoming doctor's appointments, visits to relatives, a parent being out of town, and similar events can be verbally told to your child at the same time you and he post it on his wall. Ask him if he has any questions and ask him what he thinks would make the change go easier for him.

Unpredictable changes are harder not only for your child to cope with but for you to try to help him. The first goal is to offer him empathy for his upset and try to soothe him and calm him down. Later you can talk with him about why the change was upsetting and how he thinks he can feel less upset next time.

How can my child's teacher help with insistence on routine and sameness?

Children and teens with AD function best when things are highly routine so they can predict what is going to happen throughout the day. When unexpected changes, even minor ones, occur during the school day, they tend to react with anxiety and obsessive worry, which in turn can lead to behavior problems and emotional outbursts. Try to help your child's teacher understand that you, of course, know that your child has to learn to cope with change and unexpected disruptions, but that his AD makes this far more difficult for him than the average child. His difficulty coping with change is a symptom of his AD and he will respond best with support and accommodation rather than throwing him into the changes and forcing him to deal with it. Some tips for teachers include:

- Provide a consistent daily classroom routine
- Post the daily schedule on the wall or board
- Highlight any changes on the schedule
- Announce as soon as you know of any changes
- Write changes on the wall calendar or chalkboard
- Expose child to the upcoming change if possible
- Use pictures/wall calendar to indicate changes and upcoming events

How can my child's teacher help with flexibility?

The goal at school, like at home, is flexibility. Teachers are used to preparing students for upcoming changes. They use calendars, daily announcements, and notes on the chalkboard. The real challenge comes with unpredictable changes. Teachers can set up unexpected changes that are small and ones she thinks the AD child will be able to handle. Small things such as using a different color chalk, taking roll call backwards, and having a surprise treat are small changes that can help the child experience change in a safe way. Prompting for changes in activities by counting down, such as announcing ten, five, and one minutes before the bell rings helps the child prepare himself for the upcoming change.

Your teacher can also talk about things that "might" happen. For example, begin reviewing fire drill procedures on Monday for the upcoming Friday drill. In very early elementary years, teachers have their class practice for the fire drill before it happens so that when it comes they are prepared. The AD child needs this type of preparation far longer than his peers.

How does the insistence on routine and sameness affect my child's play?

The insistence on routine and sameness interferes with the AD child's play. Not all AD children engage in repetitive play patterns, but for those who do, it can be very disruptive in play. Play for most children is free-flowing with a give and take between playmates where they each play off the other's contribution. One of the most enjoyable aspects of play is the unpredictability and uniqueness that playmates bring to the play. The AD child, however, is disturbed by the free flow of play. She has a set routine in her mind for her play and becomes frustrated when someone attempts to disrupt it. The more rigid and insistent the child is that the play goes exactly as she wants it the more social rejection she will experience.

The AD child who sticks to a rigid play routine also misses out on the joy of solitary play. Even when children play by themselves, their play is still free flowing, imaginative, and fun. The AD child's play in contrast tends to be routine and predictable and to the outside observer appears to be more of a task than play.

How do special interests affect my child's play?

There is a great overlap between the special interests and play patterns of AD children. Most commonly, the special interest dominates the AD child's play. While many children have a favorite type of toy or game they like to play, the AD child's preference is rigid and does not allow room for other interests. He only wants to play his special interest and is very resistant towards playing with anything else. If he plays with others, he is insistent that they play his special interest. He may be overprotective with his special interest collection, refusing to let his peers play with the items. His play is less physically active and playful, but more verbal where he enjoys showing off his knowledge about his special interest, almost as if he is giving a seminar and demonstration. If he is willing to allow his playmate to actually touch his items, he wants to tell him exactly what to do with them. He becomes easily frustrated when his peers' play deviates from what he wants to do. Arguments, outbursts, and refusing to continue to play are common events when the AD child plays with a peer.

What are normal play patterns?

To help determine if your child's play is problematic, it helps to know what the development of normal play looks like. As young as infancy, babies begin to interact with one another. They imitate each other's sounds, and between one and two years they try to engage one another in playful interactions. By age two to two and a half, toddlers use words to initiate others to play. They also engage in complementary play where each one performs a task to help the other, such as when one holds a doll while the other feeds it. Around this same age, toddlers spend much of their time playing alone even if there are other children around. This solitary play is the most frequent type of play for three- to four-year-olds and occupies about one-third of the play of kindergarten children. Parallel play develops next, where toddlers play with the same toys and do not influence one another's play but may interact by exchanging toys and talking about one another's play. Cooperative play develops later, where toddlers and young children play in an interactive manner, playing towards the same goal, such as building a sandcastle or playing make-believe.

What should I look for in my child's play?

All parents keep an eye on how their child plays with others, wondering if their child is interacting enough and is able to get along with age-mates. Most worrisome to parents is when they observe their child spending too much time alone and/or being aggressive with peers. For parents of toddlers and early-elementary children, it helps to know that each of the types of play coexist and play is spent in almost equal portions between solitary, parallel, and cooperative play. The *quality* of your child's play is more important as an indicator of difficulties than the *quantity* of time spent in each type of play. Your child spending a lot of time playing alone in early childhood is not necessarily problematic. However, problems are evident if he wanders aimlessly, hovers near peers but does not interact, insists on playing alone, uses repetitive meaningless movements, or does not use imagination in play. These types of play patterns become more of a concern as the child grows older. As children enter first and second grade, they spend increasing time in cooperative play. AD children, however, continue for many years to prefer to play alone and fail to engage in pretend play.

What are the play difficulties of children and teens with Asperger's Disorder?

Children with AD have great difficulties with playing with peers. They cannot participate in the give and take of play and cannot tolerate the many shifts that happen in play. They have one-sided play and become upset when the other child does not play their way. Unlike most children, who will compromise for the sake of keeping a playmate, the AD child is rigid and refuses to compromise. He has trouble playing in a group and does better one-on-one. He often chooses to play by himself, preferring not to have to accommodate another person. He finds more acceptance and tolerance when playing with older children and adults.

AD children:

- Do not know how to join other children playing
- Rigidly play the way they want to
- Lack flexibility to play with another child
- Do not play cooperatively or take turns
- Do not learn from watching other children
- Do not profit from play experiences
- Reject offers from peers to play
- Isolate themselves from peers
- Do not pay attention to their playmate
- Do not engage in imaginative or make-believe play

Why is play so important?

Psychologists have studied children for many decades and have found that early problems in play have a strong negative impact on social relationships. This is the case not only during childhood—there are lasting negative effects on adult relationships.

While play may seem to be simply a source of fun, it is actually a crucial aspect of children's development. Through play, children develop complex social skills that allow them to interact with others, form friendships, develop empathy, and resolve conflicts, skills they will use throughout their lifetime. By the end of preschool, most children have acquired complex social skills that will serve as a foundation for future relationships.

These early skills are displayed in cooperative play, an advanced form of play that involves sophisticated cognitive, emotional, and social skills where the children must respond to one another's actions, words, and behavior. Emotions are a large part of cooperative play, and children must understand and respond to their playmate's feelings as well as regulate their own. They resolve differences and disputes through negation, a key skill in getting along with others.

The solitary and rigid play patterns of AD children interfere with the natural course of using play to develop proper social skills.

How do I know if my child has play problems?

The AD child will successfully manage parallel play during preschool years where she plays next to, but not with, another child. She prefers to play alone, and if other children do not interrupt her, this pattern may go unnoticed as a problem. However, many AD toddlers can be insistent on being alone and angrily tell others to go away by yelling, hitting, and tattling. This preference to play alone persists throughout childhood. Even though the AD child will complain that no one wants to play with him, he is not truly interested in playing "with" someone. He does not want to share his toys, thoughts, or feelings with his playmate.

Preschoolers love to play make-believe, using their imagination to enrich their play. Pretend play encompasses a large part of children's play throughout elementary school. The AD child, however, is not interested in make-believe. Non-AD children have rich themes of play filled with a story whose characters interact with one another. AD children's play looks rather dull in comparison. Toys may be organized, talked about, and moved around, but little free-flowing imagination is evident.

Should I encourage my child to play with others?

Given all the difficulties the AD child has when he plays with others, parents often ask if it might be better to simply avoid play-dates. If he plays alone, he won't have social conflicts, be rejected, or suffer frustration and anger outbursts that often occur when he has a playmate. While this is certainly true and will make life easier for you and your child in the present time, it will deprive your child of the necessary experiences to develop social skills.

You can try to teach him all the social skills in the world, but nothing can teach social skills better than direct experience playing with peers. Children learn how to get along with others by actually interacting with them, observing their reactions, and modifying their behavior to fit the situation. Through trial and error children learn what works to get along with others and what gets you rejected.

Your AD child will surely experience social problems and rejection. As difficult as it is to see this happen, it is best to resist your protective instincts to keep your child alone. Instead there are ways that you can be protective during playdates while helping him to increase his play and social skills.

How can I help my child improve play skills?

Most children enjoy playing games with their parents. You can give your child special attention while you play with him and simultaneously help him learn how to play.

Don't worry about whether or not the child is good at a particular game or play activity; the focus is not on building competence in the game but on building social skills so your child becomes a desirable playmate.

You become your child's playmate and actually play with him. Take care not to turn the play into an obvious lesson. Be subtle in your teaching, giving comments about how his words and behavior affect you as a playmate. Give occasional feedback such as, "I think we both should decide what to play," "I am getting bored with this because you are not letting me have a turn," and "I am not having much fun because you are telling me everything I have to do; it would be more fun if I can do something too." You are not teaching, but giving feedback about how he is impacting you and what you would like to have happen as a playmate. Do not insist that he comply with your feedback, just state it and let him respond.

How can playdates help improve my child's social skills?

Playdates give your child an opportunity to have fun with an age-mate. The more chances she has for fun, the more joy she will experience and the greater chance she has to learn how to experience share and coregulate.

Playdates for AD children are best when they are brief, supervised by a parent, and have a focused activity. Your child should certainly have free time to play as she wishes without being scrutinized; however, she will also need your watchful eye nearby to help direct her and her playmate how to get along and use their social skills. Until you know your child can get along well with a particular peer, it is best to help them choose an activity that can take place while you are within earshot.

Many parents experience difficulty in finding playmates for their AD child. A surefire way is to volunteer to baby-sit another child for a short period of time. There are likely other parents in your neighborhood who are experiencing the same difficulty. Not only will both parents find their child a playmate, they can take turns doing the baby-sitting while the other parent gets a few hours of free time.

What kind of activities can help my child's play skills?

The more activities you can do with your child the more he is going to learn how to interact and relate to others. It is not so important *what* you do with your child, but *how* you do it. So much of what happens in the course of the day involves interacting with others, so it is very important to behave and interact with others in ways that you hope your child will imitate. Even without planning activities with your child, she has countless learning opportunities each day.

Certain activities lend themselves very nicely to teaching the social skills that AD children struggle with. When children are involved in cooperative play, the likelihood of gaining social skills increases. They learn to share, take turns, get along, and empathize. Certain activities absolutely cannot be played unless there is cooperation. Choose games that require interaction. The most important point in choosing a game is that your child is interested in playing it. The following list is a small sample of games which require various levels of cooperation:

Cooperative Games for Two	Cooperative Games for Groups
Hand-clapping games	Red Rover
Frisbee	Ring around the Rosie
Catch	Pickle
Handball	Ball games: kickball, softball, soccer
Simon Says	Four-square
Card games	Card games
Board games	Board games
Puzzles	Freeze tag
Hide-and-Seek	Duck Duck Goose
Tennis	Tug-of-War
Rock-Paper-Scissors	Team Scavenger Hunt
Badminton	Hot Potato
Hangman	Musical Chairs
Tetherball	Twister
Tic-Tac-Toe	Mystery puzzle
Chess, Checkers, Backgammon	Marco Polo

What type of peer should my child play with?

All parents are concerned with who their child spends time with. As the parent of an AD child, your concerns are even greater. Should she play with a younger peer, older peer, one who also has AD, someone who shares his special interest, or one who is more socially skilled? When researchers have examined which type of peer best suits a child or teen with AD, they discovered several interesting findings.

AD children demonstrate better social skills when they spend time with peers who share their special interest. They also do better when they interact with peers who function at a similar level of social competence. When a child with AD spends time with a more socially skilled peer group, the other children tend to limit their interaction, politely ignore, or exclude the AD child. Placing him with more socially advanced peers seems to actually contribute to his social rejection and deprive him of social opportunities to make friends and to work on social skills.

In a one-to-one situation, if a more socially capable peer is willing to play with the AD child, the peer carries the weight of the relationship and compensates for the AD child's weaknesses. She will adapt to the AD child by letting her be in charge of the play and dominate the conversation, not asking for anything back, much the same way that we as adults accommodate children when we play with them. The same is true when the AD child plays with an older child who is more tolerant than age-mates.

While it seems logical to think the AD child would learn from watching the older and the more skilled playmate, in reality the AD child gets to use even fewer social skills because the older and more skilled peer ignores his social errors and does not pressure him to be an equal playmate. The more capable peers are also likely to quickly tire of the social incompetence of the AD child and to terminate the interaction.

In contrast, playing with a socially similar peer creates a situation where each child has to work to match the demands of the relationship. Thus, two AD children who have similar levels of social competence and share the same special interest make ideal playmates for one another.

Chapter 8

LANGUAGE, MOTOR SKILLS, AND SENSORY SENSITIVITY

- What is the development of language for children with Asperger's Disorder?
- What are the problems in pragmatics seen in children and teens with Asperger's Disorder?
- What are the conversation errors children and teens with Asperger's Disorder make?
- How can I help my child with pragmatics?
- How do I teach my child to start conversations?
- How do I teach my child how to keep a conversation going?
- How do I teach my child to greet others?
- How do I get my child to stop interrupting?
- What are the semantic problems children with Asperger's Disorder have?
- How do I help my child with semantics?
- What are the prosody problems Asperger's Disorder children and teens have?
- What are the motor skills problems seen in children and teens with Asperger's Disorder?
- How can I help my child with motor skills problems?
- What is auditory sensitivity?
- How can I help my child with auditory sensitivity?
- What is tactile sensitivity?
- What is gustatory sensitivity?
- What are visual and olfactory sensitivities?

What is the development of language for children with Asperger's Disorder?

Approximately 50 percent of children with AD have delayed speech. However, once speech starts, it typically progresses rapidly. By age five, they should have caught up to their peers. Whether or not an AD child's speech is delayed, the majority of children with AD nonetheless experience language difficulties. AD children have a very unique way of talking that others perceive as a bit peculiar. Their conversation, choice of words, pronunciation, and/or tone may be unusual. Speech therapists use a specific vocabulary to define the language problems of AD children, and break the problems into three categories:

- Pragmatics: how language is used
- Semantics: the meaning of words
- Prosody: the pitch, rhythm, and stress placed on words

Problems in pragmatics manifest in odd ways of conversing with others. Semantic problems result in literal interpretation of words. Prosody problems give an odd quality to the way the child sounds as he talks. These three areas result in numerous problems with language and the way AD children and teens speak to others.

What are the problems in pragmatics seen in children and teens with Asperger's Disorder?

Pragmatics refers to how one uses language. Children and teens with AD have difficulties using language to communicate. Their errors in pragmatics cause social challenges because of their trouble relating to others though conversation. There are numerous conversational errors, including:

- Interrupts others
- Dominates conversations
- Talks about topics others show no interest in
- Makes little eye contact
- Has little variety in topics
- Does not take turns talking
- Ends conversations abruptly
- Does not respond to what others are saying
- Gives too much information about a topic
- Does not pause to let others join in
- Oblivious to listener's reaction
- Does not use facial expressions
- Gives long-winded monologues
- Does not request information from others
- Asks incessant questions
- Does not use people's names to initiate conversation
- Has one-sided conversations

- Does not greet others prior to starting a conversation
- Forces their topic in conversations
- Does not modify the conversation to fit the listener's interest
- Has trouble telling a story in a coherent manner
- Asks highly specific questions
- Starts conversations with odd questions
- Fails to seek clarification when confused
- Will not admit he does not know something
- Assumes others know what he knows
- Does not modify the level of detail to match the listener's knowledge
- Does not observe boredom in the listener

What are the conversational errors children and teens with Asperger's Disorder make?

Conversing with a child or teen with AD can be rather difficult. Parents of AD children may get used to their child's unusual style of talking and therefore fail to recognize the severity. They may become accustomed to rescuing their AD child from conversational errors by speaking for her, explaining to others what she meant to say, and interpreting for her. To the outside observer, however, the AD child's style of speaking is quickly seen as unusual.

A brief interaction with an AD child starts off problematic. The child does not say hello or look the other person in the eye. Regardless of the age difference and level of familiarity with the other person, she will begin the encounter by launching immediately into talking, usually about her special interest or asking an odd question that seems to come out of nowhere. She may give a nonstop monologue, not letting the other person to join in. Once the listener gets a chance to speak, the AD child disregards what he has to say, does not respond, and gets right back to where she left off.

How can I help my child with pragmatics?

Given the numerous conversation problems experienced by the AD child, this will be a long-term goal requiring patience and ongoing effort. Your child will make many errors in conversation on a daily basis, providing ample opportunity to help him. However, if you try to help him with every error he makes, you will overwhelm him. One way to approach the large number of conversational errors is to pick one skill per week to work on. Ignore the other conversational errors and provide prompting, encouragement, teaching, and praising for only the selected skill. Because his conversational problems are part of his disorder and not due to simply not knowing the skills, your expectations must be realistic. Do not expect that you will work on a skill for one week or even one month and your child will learn it and do it from that point on. Rather, a more realistic goal is to increase the number of times he uses appropriate conversation skills. Your gentle and patient encouragement over the years will raise his overall level of conversation skills so he communicates better with others throughout his life.

How do I teach my child to start conversations?

Most children do not have to be taught in detail how to start a conversation. They learn simply by being in conversations with others, watching others, and paying attention to what has worked for them in the past. AD children seem oblivious to this natural learning and need to be told exactly how to start a conversation.

With AD children so focused on their special interest, chances are many of their conversations will start off with a question or comment related to their favorite topic. When your child learns from your repeated instruction that this is not an appropriate way to begin a conversation, he may be able to restrain himself but feel anxious because he does not know what to say instead. You can teach him appropriate conversation starters that are likely to work with different people. Be sure to explain that conversations should begin with a greeting and an opening that the listener can respond to.

For example:

- Grandparents: "Hi, Grandma, it's nice to see you!"
- Child you want to play with: "Hi, can I play with you?"
- Teacher: "Good morning! How are you today?"
- Friend: "Hi, what have you been up to?"

How do I teach my child how to keep a conversation going?

AD children often do well learning how to start a conversation. They are good at memorizing exact conversation starters and with your prompts are likely to use them. Because conversations are unpredictable and cannot be memorized, AD children experience far greater struggles keeping the conversation going after they give their starter line.

Since your child will not naturally learn how to converse through experience alone, you will have to instruct her. You do not need to have any formal instruction, but rather simply through conversing with your child, you gain ample opportunity to teach communication skills. If you can help your child with the two most important skills in conversing, you will greatly improve her ability to carry on conversations. Focus on encouraging your child to:

- "Listen to what I say."
- "Say something about what I just said."

In conversation, if your child responds to you with a completely unrelated statement, gently remind her, "Honey, I just said that I loved the pizza we had last night, and you asked me what type of engine 747 airplanes have. Can you say something about my pizza comment before you change the subject to airplanes?" You are nicely describing to her what was incorrect and what she needs to do to keep the conversation on track.

How do I teach my child to greet others?

Young children need to be taught to appropriately greet others, but eventually do this on their own without prompting. AD children, however, fail to do so well into their teen and even adult years. Even children who have been in social skills groups for years still need weekly reminders to say hello to the other group members. When they comply, it is with a monotone one-word greeting. They simply are not interested in the social niceties and it is very hard for them to grasp the idea that even if they do not like to do it, it is part of how we relate to one another. They do not understand that their failure to greet others or their flat facial expression and robotic "hello" is what quickly makes others judge them negatively. You will therefore have to teach the lesson of greeting others for many years. Prompt your child to say hello to others and remind him of each step he needs to include:

- Look the person in the eye
- Smile
- Say "Hello, Dr. Marshall" in a friendly voice
- Keep looking the person in the eye
- Listen to person say hello back to you

How do I get my child to stop interrupting?

Most children and teens interrupt far more often than their parents care for. Parents find it takes years of reminders before their child eventually learns to consistently wait his turn to talk. The AD child, however, keeps interrupting despite years of instruction because he fails to read the signals of when it is his turn to talk.

You can decrease the interruptions by creating a set of code words and/or hand signals to let him know when he needs to wait to talk and when it is okay.

- Red light: No talking right now; wait until I give you a green light
- Yellow light: No talking right now, but if you wait, it will just be about a minute
- Green light: It is now your turn to talk

Teach your child that you will employ the light system so that you do not have to raise your voice to him when he interrupts, which will be far more pleasant for both of you. Explain to him what each light means. Expect that you will have to work at this because he will have countless moments when he believes what he has to say is so important that it simply cannot wait!

What are the semantic problems children with Asperger's Disorder have?

Semantics refers to the meaning of words. Despite the finding that most children and teens with AD have advanced verbal skills, most also have trouble with semantics, including:

- Pedantic speech
- Literal interpretation
- Difficulty understanding sarcasm
- Difficulty understanding figures of speech
- Misinterpretation of teasing as intentional insults
- Difficulty understanding humor and jokes
- Inability to understand metaphors
- Inability to understand double entendres

Some AD children speak with a confusing mix of pedantic speech that is overly precise, highly formal, and too advanced for most of their peers to understand. They may speak more like a brilliant adult than a child or adolescent, leading some to refer to AD as "the little professor" syndrome. AD children have no fear of correcting adults who use words they find to be less-than-perfect for the sentence.

In contrast to their advanced verbal expression, AD children and teens are often confused by language. They often have a poor sense of humor and do not understand teasing or sarcasm. They interpret things literally and therefore also misunderstand figures of speech. Hearing "if looks could kill" may result in the child asking if looks can really kill someone.

How do I help my child with semantics?

Through ordinary communication, you will be able to interpret misunderstandings for your child. It will not always be easy to tell when your child is confused, and he will be unlikely to openly declare his need for help. You can interpret words, phrases, metaphors, and figures of speech for him.

To help with figures of speech, your child will probably enjoy making a book with drawings or magazine pictures, one picture to illustrate the literal meaning and one for the real meaning. Your child is sure to have fun making silly pictures of "cat got your tongue?" or "the early bird gets the worm" and then finding pictures that show the correct meaning. Children's joke books and comedies can increase understanding of humor.

The most difficult challenge will be in helping your child understand teasing and sarcasm, as he will interpret these literally and miss the emotional tone and intention. You can help him by prompting him to think about who is teasing, is the tone of their voice friendly, are they smiling, and what happened just before the teasing or sarcasm. In this way he can come to interpret the intent of the words, instead of only their exact definition.

What are the prosody problems children and teens with Asperger's Disorder have?

Prosody refers to the stress one places on words and the intonation. It includes how fast someone talks, how loud he is, how he pronounces words, and how rhythmic his speech is.

Prosody problems include:

- Loud talking
- Overly precise pronunciation
- Unusual rhythm when talking
- Lack of inflection
- Absence of emotion in voice
- Monotonous sound
- Stilted or halted speech
- Difficulty coordinating breathing while talking

Children and teens with AD generally have multiple problems with prosody. The manner in which they speak is unusual. They lack a smooth flow and rhythm to their speech. Some speak in a robotic-like manner with no emphasis on any words. Their pace does not vary and they show little emotion in their words. Some have halted or stilted speech, almost as if their words are being interrupted by their breathing. They can be monotone and dull to listen to. Their pronunciation can be exaggerated, where they slowly pronounce each syllable.

While pragmatics and semantics are specialties that often require the help of a speech therapist, problems with prosody most certainly do. Speech therapy will teach your child techniques that require the skill of a speech and language expert.

What are the motor skills problems seen in children and teens with Asperger's Disorder?

Motor skills weakness is commonly seen in children and teens with AD. It is estimated that 50–90 percent of children with AD have motor skills problems.

You may have observed problems in some of the following motor skills:

Locomotion: Walking and running gaits may appear unusual. This will interfere with basic childhood play of games such as tag and hide-and-seek. Children's locomotion problems are visually apparent to their peers, and they may be called clumsy or klutzy and are easy targets for teasing. They are also likely to be the last chosen for teams.

Ball skills: Catching and throwing are poor. Children with motor skills problems fail to watch the ball when trying to catch it; they raise their hands too late and position them too wide or too narrow. Kicking a ball is poor. Poor ball skills translate into teasing, criticism, and rejection, as peers are angered when the AD child causes them to lose a game.

Balance: Balancing on one leg can be problematic and cause problems with hopscotch and jumping rope. This has less impact on play and team activities than locomotion and ball skills.

Manual dexterity: Also called fine motor movement, manual dexterity is the ability to use the hands to manipulate objects. Skills such as writing, coloring, cutting with scissors, buttoning clothing, and tying shoes can be challenges for children with AD. Handwriting can be the cause of many behavior problems. Procrastination, disrupting the classroom, and tantrumming may be seen as tactics the AD child uses to avoid writing.

Coordination: This refers to the control of the body in sync with the arms and legs. Skills such as riding a bike and Rollerblading are achieved quite late for many children with AD.

Rhythm: Some children have trouble with rhythm. This may result in trouble with rhythmic motions such as clapping to a beat.

How can I help my child with motor skills problems?

An occupational or physiotherapist is the appropriate professional to evaluate your child's motor skills. In addition to general observation, there are standardized tests an occupational therapist will use to determine if your child has motor skills weaknesses.

Occupational Therapy, OT for short, is designed to help with fine and gross motor skills. Fine motor skills training helps children with small movements of the hands to manipulate objects to aid with handwriting or buttoning clothing. Gross motor skills training addresses large body movements and helps children gain better control of their body.

You may be surprised to find that if your child has trouble printing or writing that the therapy does not actually involve practicing these skills, but instead includes a variety of activities designed to strengthen the same muscles used in writing. OT may appear to be just playing, and parents observing their child digging beans out of Play-Doh or jumping over blocks may wonder why they need to pay a professional to play with their child. Rest assured, OT has well-researched techniques that help build fine and gross motor skills.

What is auditory sensitivity?

AD children can have sensitivity to certain sounds. Sudden, unexpected loud noises can be particularly irritating, and the AD child with auditory sensitivity will overreact. Barking dogs, alarm clocks, and loud speakers may be upsetting. Noises from motors such as a lawn mower or hair-dryer can be very irritating. Multiple simultaneous noises also can spark a reaction. Children may be upset by noises in crowds, sudden noises, sirens, and alarms. Reactions such as covering their ears with their hands are often seen. More upsetting reactions seen may be agitation or anger that causes an outburst or emotional shutdown where your child simply refuses to move or talk. Even the classroom with the background noise can be agitating to the AD child. While most people can screen out background noise, children with AD have great trouble doing so.

Few people can relate to these noises being worthy of much reaction; however, if one imagines that these noises are akin to nails being scratched on a chalkboard, it is easier to empathize with the AD child's aversion to particular noises. AD children have trouble ignoring, tuning out, and not reacting to these types of noises.

How can I help my child with auditory sensitivity?

If your child is sensitive to noises, you probably already have noticed it. Watch his reaction to various noises and keep notes of what seems to upset him and what appears to calm him down. He may not be aware that certain noises bother him. You may see obvious signs such as him running out of the room, putting his hands over his ears, crying, screaming, or crawling under a table. Some children may not be so obvious in their reaction and may display their upset in behaviors that are not so easy to connect to a particular noise. Your child may display a sudden outburst of anger, argue with or hit his sibling, or begin to act up. Taking notes on his behavior and what was happening before it will help you discover patterns of what sets him off.

If the kitchen blender does not bother him, then there is nothing to change. However, if he begins to argue with his brother every time you use the blender, take note that this might be irritating him. Remove, limit, or decrease the sound level of noises that are in your control.

- Turn down telephone ringers.
- Replace doorbell with door knocker.
- Limit using noisy kitchen equipment when your child is at home.
- Avoid noisy, crowded situations.
- Schedule noisy workmen (e.g., gardener, construction) when your child is not home.

For noises that you can anticipate but cannot stop or control, use preparation to help decrease a reaction. Use a plan of warn and distract. Warn him of the noise that will be made, and set him up with a distracting activity. If you know that blow-drying your hair causes your child irritation, set him up in another room with a pleasurable activity and tell him that you will be using the blow-dryer and you know he does not like the noise so he should try to stay out of your bathroom until you are done.

Some ways to distract your child from noises include:

- Watch a DVD
- Play a video game
- Listen to music with headphones
- Listen to a book on tape with headphones
- Go to another room in the house
- Play outside
- Use earplugs
- Use noise-reducing headphones in noisy places such as airports, airplanes, buses

What is tactile sensitivity?

Tactile refers to the sensation of touch. Some AD children are overly sensitive to being touched. They react with stiffening and physically withdrawing from hugs, kisses, and pats of affection. Occupational therapists call this type of physical backing away tactile defensiveness. AD children can also be sensitive to physical sensations that come from objects. Tags inside shirts, elastic around the ankles in socks, and stiff or itchy fabrics seem to be particularly bothersome.

Occupational therapists advise that children with tactile sensitivity and tactile defensiveness be treated with a combination of accommodation and exposure.

Accommodation involves providing your child with the type of touch he prefers and initially avoiding the type he does not like. Purchasing the type of clothing he is comfortable in helps decrease daily upsets. Some AD children's wardrobes consist of sweatsuits with the tags cut out, bootie-style socks, and slip-on shoes. Gradual exposure to other types of touch and other types of fabric slowly allows the AD child to experience touch and fabrics that irritate him. Occupational therapists introduce various types of touch and materials in a play-like setting. Parents participate under the occupational therapist's guidance in exposing their child to the stimulation.

What is gustatory sensitivity?

Gustatory refers to taste. Some AD children have strong aversions to certain foods.

The sensitivity may be due to taste, smell, or texture. They may refuse to eat all but a few select items. Ordinarily refusing to cater to a child's picky eating habits results in him learning that if he does not eat what is served, he will not eat until the next meal. AD children can have such strong aversions that they will simply refuse to eat, regardless of how hungry they are, until they are given their preferred food. Forcing an AD child to eat certain foods or withholding food until he eats what you serve him is therefore not a recommended approach. Most AD children eventually outgrow gustatory sensitivity but may still have a somewhat restricted range of preferred foods. Consultation with your child's pediatrician and/or a referral to a pediatric nutritionist may be necessary to ensure that your child is getting proper nutrients.

Therapy for gustatory sensitivity is usually not necessary unless a child is failing to gain weight, is losing weight, is having frequent episodes of refusing to eat, has extreme reactions to foods, or shows problems with chewing and/or swallowing food. Consultation with an occupational therapist can determine if therapy is needed.

What are visual and olfactory sensitivities?

Visual sensitivity is a discomfort with what is seen. The most common visual sensitivity is to light. AD children can be overreactive to bright, fluorescent, neon, and flashing lights. Avoidance of bothersome lights can be difficult. You can control the lighting in your house by removing all fluorescent lights and purchasing three-way bulbs to accommodate varying preferences of family members. Allowing your child to pick out sunglasses to wear in the car can help decrease sensitivity to the bright sun. Tinted shades on the rear windows can keep the bright sunlight minimized as well.

Olfactory is the sensation of smell. Some AD children and teens can be very sensitive to smells in the environment. When they are aware of aromas they do not like, they can be rather insensitive to feelings of others and made impulsive comments such as, "Your house stinks!" Other aromas may not be obvious to your child that they are irritating to him. He may complain of headaches or show mood changes.

As with the other types of sensory sensitivities, it helps to keep a watchful eye on mood and behavior changes and see if there are any links to aromas. If your child complains about certain smells or you observe patterns related to smell, it can be helpful to try to eliminate them when possible.

Chapter 9

SUCCEEDING IN SCHOOL

- Should I tell my child's teacher about his or her Asperger's Disorder?
- Do children with Asperger's Disorder qualify for special education?
- What is Section 504?
- Who qualifies for Section 504?
- What is a Section 504 meeting?
- What are reasonable accommodations under Section 504?
- What should I do if my child is denied Section 504?
- What is the IDEA 2004 law for special education?
- Who qualifies for special education under IDEA 2004?
- What steps are necessary to obtain special education under IDEA 2004?
- What tests are included in the evaluation for special education?
- What is an IEP?
- What should be included in the written IEP?
- What special education services are available?
- What if my child is denied special education services under IDEA?
- Can children with Asperger's Disorder be denied special education?
- Will the school accept an independent assessment?
- What are parents' responsibilities in the special education process?
- How can a special education advocate help?
- What if my child's school does not have special education?
- What if my child goes to a private school?
- Will special education stigmatize my child?
- What should I know about my child's special education records?
- Who can access my child's records?
- What are the exceptions to the privacy of my child's records?
- How can I find out how my child is doing in the classroom?
- Should my child repeat a grade to give him time to mature?
- How are behavior problems handled through special education?
- How are suspensions and expulsions handled for special education students?

Should I tell my child's teacher about his or her Asperger's Disorder?

At the beginning of the new school year, parents and children are optimistic that the child will have a fresh start. Parents wonder if they should tell the new teacher that their child has AD, questioning if knowing the child has a disorder will bias the teacher against their child. They hold out hope that the fresh start will last and if the teacher is not aware of the disorder, the child's problems will not be discovered.

Unfortunately, this rarely happens. Children cannot hide their AD. The symptoms are certain to show after the initial honeymoon phase of the new school year is over. Not telling the teacher leaves her to guess what is causing the child's difficulties.

Rather than blindsiding the teacher, you can be far more helpful to her and to your child by informing her right up front. A note to the teacher indicating that your child has AD and a request to meet with her in the first few weeks of school is suggested. Prepare information for the meeting, providing the teacher with a list of behaviors she is likely to observe in your child and a list of proposed solutions that you and prior teachers have found helpful.

Do children with Asperger's Disorder qualify for special education?

Children and teens with AD do qualify for special education. AD is now the sixth most commonly classified disability in special education. In fact, the number of students classified as AD has increased six fold since 1994. This increase is due to AD being added to the *DSM-IV-TR* as a new disorder and the change of allowing autism to be diagnosed in people with a normal IQ. Prior to 1994, students with an IQ above 70 were not considered to have autism and would not have qualified for special education under the autism classification.

Two federal laws, Section 504 and IDEA, now guarantee children with AD a "free appropriate public education" in the "least restrictive environment." Free means the education must be of no cost to the parents and appropriate means that it must meet the individual needs of each child. The least restrictive environment means that children with disabilities are not to be segregated from their nondisabled peers simply because of their disability. If they are to be removed from their peers, it is only for the portion of their education that cannot be met in the general or mainstream classroom.

Each law has different procedures and criteria for eligibility and different services available. IDEA states that the child must have a disability that requires special education services. Section 504 has a lower threshold and requires only that the child need modifications and accommodations in order to take part in learning. All public schools across the nation that receive federal funds are required to follow these two federal laws.

What is Section 504?

Section 504 is the section of the Rehabilitation Act of 1973 that applies to persons with disabilities. It is a civil rights act that protects the civil rights of persons with disabilities including AD. It also protects students with disabilities from harassment. For practical purposes, what Section 504 means to you is that public schools cannot discriminate against your child and must make "reasonable accommodations and modifications" for his disability. It is designed to level the playing field for individuals with disabilities and to ensure that they have the same access to learning that individuals without disabilities have.

For most students with AD, the reason to obtain Section 504 is that the child does not need a special education setting but is in need of accommodations and modifications in order to be successful in school. Section 504 makes allowances, modifications, and/or accommodations to help the child with AD compensate in areas where their disorder causes a significant negative impact on their educational performance.

Children who have AD but do not meet criteria under IDEA are often eligible for assistance under Section 504. If a child is qualified under IDEA, he is automatically qualified under Section 504; however, the reverse is not true.

Who qualifies for Section 504?

A student is eligible for Section 504 if he meets the definition of a "qualified handicapped person." The student does not need to be eligible for special education under IDEA in order to be a "handicapped person" or to be protected and provided accommodations and modifications under Section 504. To qualify for Section 504, the child must:

- Be determined to have a physical or mental impairment that substantially limits one or more major life activities, including learning and behavior
- Have a record of having such an impairment, or
- Be regarded as having such an impairment

In addition to a wide variety of physical disabilities and mental disorders, AD is included in this legal definition. The term *major life activities* includes learning and, therefore, applies to the school setting.

Not every student with AD will qualify for Section 504. Their AD must be determined to substantially limit their learning. The school district is required, if requested by the parents, to determine if the child's AD is substantially limiting his success in school. However, the evaluation is not required to be a full evaluation simply because a parent requests one. The school is allowed to determine that a pre-screening meets the criteria for an evaluation.

What is a Section 504 meeting?

A Section 504 meeting is between parents and school personnel to discuss the child's eligibility for accommodations and modifications. The school may initiate the meeting after identifying the child as having a potential disability that is interfering with learning. However, more often than not, the parents identify the difficulties their child is having due to a disability.

Parents can request a Section 504 meeting to determine eligibility for accommodations and modifications by writing to the school principal. Once the meeting is scheduled, parents are invited to attend and take part along with the child's teachers and any school personnel familiar with the child.

Be prepared to present your case for why your child needs accommodations and modifications. A report from your child's pediatrician or psychologist documenting his diagnosis should be brought to the meeting. Bring a list of your child's behaviors and how they impair his learning. While you are not obligated to come up with solutions, having a list of suggestions will be very helpful and will increase your child's chances of obtaining the highest number of necessary accommodations and modifications.

If your child is determined to be eligible under Section 504, the regulations require that there be a written plan that describes what those accommodations and modifications will be.

What are reasonable accommodations under Section 504?

As recipients of federal funding, under Section 504 public schools must make "reasonable" accommodations and modifications for the eligible child unless they can demonstrate that to do so would impose an undue hardship on the operation of their program. Accommodations and modifications should be designed to place the student who has a disability at an equal starting level with the non-handicapped student.

For AD children, Section 504 has been a saving grace, allowing the child to remain in the general education classroom but be accommodated to ease their struggles. Some examples of accommodations and modifications for the AD child in the main categories of impairment include:

- Insistence on Routine:
    Prepare in advance for change
    Post rules on wall
- Sensory Sensitivity:
    Allow use of earplugs
    Offer alternative activities
- Socialization:
    Pair student with a supportive buddy
    Monitor closely on playground
- Organization and Planning:
    Keep second set of textbooks at home
    Provide assignment book
- Compliance:
    Post rules in classroom
    Maintain behavior-modification system in the classroom
- Mood:
    Compliment positive behavior
    Focus on student's talents
- Fine Motor Coordination:
    Allow use of computer
    Provide extra time on writing tasks

What should I do if my child is denied Section 504?

Perhaps one of the most frustrating aspects of advocating for your child's education is to see each day how he struggles in school, only to be informed that he does not meet criteria for eligibility.

Impairment, in and of itself, does not qualify your child for protection under Section 504. The impairment must substantially limit one or more major life activities in order to qualify for Section 504. Under Section 504, your child must not only have at least one disorder, but that disorder must negatively influence his ability to learn and/or perform academically.

If you believe your child meets criteria for Section 504 and he has been denied accommodations and modifications, you have a right to appeal this decision to the school. Each school district has its own appeal process. You can begin the appeal process by asking your child's school for a printed copy of the district's policies and procedures for Section 504. This written document may be titled "Policies, Procedures, Safeguards, Parental Rights," or a similar name. The appeal process should be outlined in the written document and it should be relatively easy for you to appeal the denial.

What is the IDEA 2004 law for special education?

IDEA 2004 is the federal law that governs special education services. IDEA 2004 stands for Individuals with Disabilities Education Improvement Act of 2004 (IDEA 2004 for short). This law protects students who need special education due to a disability. The law states that a child is entitled to a Free and Appropriate Education (FAPE) in the "least restrictive environment." To the greatest extent possible, the child protected by IDEA 2004 is to be educated in the mainstream classroom. IDEA 2004 thus prevents children with disabilities from being unnecessarily segregated from their nondisabled peers.

Under IDEA 2004, children who are identified as having a potential disability are entitled to an evaluation at the school district's expense. Either a teacher or parent may identify the child as having a potential disability. Parents knowing or suspecting their child has AD is not sufficient to require the school to perform an evaluation; the disorder must have an adverse effect on "educational performance." Educational performance refers to much more than your child's grades. It encompasses your child's complete functioning in all aspects of school, including his ability to behave, get along with peers, and complete work, among many other things.

Who qualifies for special education under IDEA 2004?

To qualify under IDEA 2004, children must meet three requirements. First they must be between the ages of three and twenty-one years and not yet graduated from high school. Second, they must have at least one of the eligible specific disabilities listed under IDEA 2004. Third, they must require special education because of that disability.

Simply having a disability does not make someone eligible for services. The child must have a need for services because of the disability. Many children with AD, despite having the disorder, do not have their educational performance or school behavior affected by it. Such children would not be eligible for special education services under IDEA 2004.

The eligible disabilities are limited to:

- Autism (includes AD)
- Hearing impairments including deafness
- Mental retardation
- Multiple disabilities

- Orthopedic impairments
- Emotional disturbance
- Specific learning disabilities
- Speech or language impairments
- Traumatic brain injuries
- Visual impairments including blindness
- Other health impairments (includes ADHD)

Children with AD who qualify under IDEA 2004 are likely to have a history of significant problems with completing class work, following rules, disrupting the class, and conflicts with peers, among others.

What steps are necessary to obtain special education under IDEA 2004?

If you believe your child is in need of special education services, send a written request for an evaluation to the school principal. Each state sets its own period in which the school must respond to your request. For example, in California the school has fifteen calendar days to respond. Once parental consent is given for the assessment, the school then has sixty calendar days to complete it. Parents should check their state department of education website to determine the period in which their school must respond and evaluate.

Your child's school will either deny your request to assess or invite you to attend an "assessment" or "student study team" meeting. The meeting takes place to discuss the rationale and need for an assessment. If an assessment is granted, you will receive a written assessment plan, which you are to review and sign to consent that the assessment take place. Some schools will skip the meeting and directly send you a written assessment plan.

An assessment will likely include:

- Individually administered standardized academic achievement tests
- Teacher observations
- Review of classroom performance
- Speech and language assessment
- Social-emotional assessment
- Cognitive ability/intelligence assessment

What tests are included in the evaluation for special education?

Typically, the school psychologist will select a battery of tests to measure various areas of a child's functioning. Additional specialists will administer tests that are outside the realm of academics and behavior. A speech pathologist will use speech and language tests. A nurse will screen for vision and hearing deficits. An occupational therapist will assess fine and gross motor functioning.

Behavioral functioning is assessed by standardized questionnaires completed by parents and the teacher. Academic achievement is assessed by a standardized test administered face-to-face to measure the grade level achieved by your child in a wide variety of academic skills.

In order to evaluate for a specific learning disorder, a child's intellectual/cognitive ability must be measured. Some schools achieve this by administering an IQ test. However, decades ago, a court ruling found that IQ tests discriminated against African American children and resulted in too many African American students being inappropriately placed in special education based solely on IQ, causing most schools to abandon IQ tests. While nothing legally prohibits schools from using IQ tests to determine intelligence, most schools opt to use alternative tests to estimate cognitive ability.

School psychologists do not use test data to make a diagnosis of any disorder or disability. Results are used solely to determine eligibility, placement, and goals.

What is an IEP?

Once your child has been assessed by the school, you will be invited to attend the IEP meeting. IEP stands for Individualized Education Plan. In this meeting, you will meet with school personnel to discuss the assessment results and determine if your child is eligible for special education under IDEA 2004. The invitation to the IEP must be given at least ten days in advance and scheduled at a mutually convenient time for the parents and school personnel. Parents have a right to reschedule the IEP if necessary.

The IEP meeting must include:

- Parent or legal guardian
- Teacher who is familiar with the student
- General education teacher
- Special education teacher
- School professional(s) who is qualified to explain the test data
- School representative who is able to authorize special education

If your child is eligible for special education, an IEP will be written. The school is obligated to provide only what is documented in the IEP. Do not accept a verbal promise of anything related to your child's education. You may take the IEP home with you to review. Carefully read the IEP and sign it only when you agree it is appropriate for your child's education. If you do not agree to a small part of the IEP, you may ask your school if they have an informal dispute resolution, where minor disagreements can be quickly settled. If your school does not have such a process or if you are in disagreement with the IEP as a whole, your next step is to file for due process, a formal process where you will have mediation and/or a hearing in order to resolve the disagreement.

What should be included in the written IEP?

In addition to the IEP meeting, an IEP is also a written document that describes the educational, developmental, and behavioral support the child with a disability will receive. The school must supply what is written in the IEP. Contrarily, if it is not written in the IEP, the school does not have to provide it. An IEP must include:

- The child's specific eligibility for special education
- The child's present level of educational performance and how his disability affects his involvement and progress in the general curriculum
- Measurable goals to meet the child's needs, enabling him to be involved in and progress with the general curriculum
- A statement of the special education and related services and supplemental aids and services
- Placement, with a description of the educational placement as the least restrictive environment
- Program accommodations and modifications or supports for the school personnel that will be provided for the child to advance appropriately toward attaining the annual goals
- An explanation of the extent to which the child will not participate with nondisabled children in the regular class

The IEP is reviewed annually to reestablish eligibility, evaluate progress, and make any necessary modifications.

What special education services are available?

Special education is to be provided in the least restrictive environment. This means that your child should be educated in the general education classroom to the furthest extent possible. The range of special education placements includes full inclusion in the regular classroom; resource specialist program, where your child may go to a specialized classroom for a particular subject or receive this service in a collaborative setting; and special day class, where the child is educated for the most part with other disabled students or only with disabled students.

In addition to placement, there is also a variety of related services (in California called Designated Instructional Services or DIS) available under IDEA 2004. Your child will be provided only the related services deemed necessary for a Free and Appropriate Education (FAPE). Some of the available services include:

- Assistive technology
- Speech therapy
- Occupational therapy
- Educational therapy
- Counseling
- Medical services
- Parent counseling and training
- Physical therapy
- Transportation
- Psychological services

In a few very severe cases where a child cannot receive a FAPE, he may qualify for a nonpublic school. These schools provide specialized services for children with specific disabilities. In the most extreme cases where a child is not safe in the home due to her disability and therefore cannot receive a FAPE while remaining at home, residential placement may be available.

What if my child is denied special education services under IDEA 2004?

Children can be denied special education under IDEA 2004 at various points in the process. Your request for an evaluation may be denied. Your child may be evaluated but found ineligible. Or, you may not agree with the goals, objectives, services, or placement the school offers.

Parents may appeal a denial. However, a denial is unlikely to be overturned without evidence that your child's AD has an adverse effect on his educational performance, including grades, achievement test scores, behavior problems, impaired or inappropriate social relations, or impaired work skills.

The first step in appealing the school's denial is to informally request a meeting with an official from the school district to discuss your child's eligibility. If this is not successful, the next step is to file for a due process hearing.

A due process hearing is a formal legal process that varies from state to state. Details on how to file and what steps to take are spelled out in a document provided by each school district, usually entitled "Procedurals Safeguards." The hearing procedure will involve the filing of motions, presentation of evidence, and possible testimony. You should not attempt to file for a due process hearing without an attorney.

Can children with Asperger's Disorder be denied special education?

It is not uncommon for schools to deny special education services for children with AD. Many children do not even get approved for an evaluation. Schools may justify their denial of services by citing the fact that the child is of average or above IQ and has no apparent learning disorder based upon her standardized academic achievement scores. Since most children with AD are of average or above IQ and only a small percent have a diagnosable learning disorder, the majority of parents raising AD children will face this frustrating battle.

Parents of AD children know that their child is struggling in school, no matter how intelligent the child is. The child passing his classes is often more a reflection of his parents' persistence and dedication than the child's effort, knowledge, and performance. Some schools may fail to recognize the invisible, immeasurable disorder of AD and may not view it as a disability that requires special assistance.

The best way to combat this unjustified denial of services is to know the criteria for services under IDEA 2004 and Section 504. If your child meets the criteria, then she is eligible, and the school must obey the law and provide services.

Will the school accept an independent assessment?

While schools are required to consider outside sources of information about your child, they are not mandated to agree with it. Even if you have a private evaluation, your child's school will conduct their own evaluation.

There are benefits to seeking an independent assessment. It can be done quickly, in comparison to the school district's waiting period. It is also likely to be more thorough than the assessment done by the school. An IQ test can be administered, which provides far more information than the alternative tests most schools will use to estimate IQ. You will also be provided with a detailed written report of the test scores and findings that your evaluator will explain to you in a face-to-face meeting. The only downside to a private evaluation is the cost that you may bear, which can range from $1,000 to $3,000 or more.

Your private evaluator may reach a more complete or different understanding of your child's disability than found by the school personnel. However, if your child is determined to be eligible for special education, it is not so important that school personnel agree with your evaluator. On the other hand, if your private evaluation indicates that your child qualifies for special education but the school denies eligibility, you may appeal the denial.

What are parents' responsibilities in the special education process?

As a parent, you must play an active role in your child's education. With increasing numbers of children undergoing evaluation for special education, it is more important than ever that parents become informed about the evaluation process, services available, and their rights. Gone are the days for parents to simply turn their child's education over to the school. Some schools are excellent sources of information about special education, while others are sorely lacking. It is up to parents to stay informed and advocate for their child's needs.

Being active in your child's education includes keeping thorough records. Make a file for each year of your child's education. Place report cards, annual academic achievement test scores, notes from teachers, IEPs, Section 504 accommodation plans, and any additional records regarding your child's education in this file. Document all phone calls you have with any school personnel. Organized and complete records will be invaluable in your annual IEP and Section 504 accommodation meeting.

You are also responsible for keeping in frequent communication with your child's teacher. Going to the teacher with a teamwork approach will be well received. A "how can I help you help my child?" approach usually sets the stage for a cooperative relationship.

How can a special education advocate help?

The special education process is unknown territory for most parents. Parents are at a disadvantage in the school meetings where the policies, procedures, laws, and language of special education are known to every committee member except them. While some schools are very helpful with the special education procedures, others withhold information, leaving parents feeling lost.

For every parent who is able to obtain special education for her child on her own, another is unsuccessful. Too many parents decide they can go it alone and figure they will spend the money for an advocate if things do not turn out their way. This can be penny-wise and pound-foolish. Saving the money by not hiring an advocate costs your child another year of not getting her educational needs meet.

Parents can best obtain special education by seeking consult before the 504 or IEP meeting with a special education advocate. These specialists know the special education laws. They know the school district personnel, what services are available, how to interpret the assessment results, and can advise you regarding your child's needs. They accompany you to the school meetings, speak on your behalf, and are very successful at getting your child the services he needs.

What if my child's school does not have special education?

Federal law requires that children who qualify for special education be provided access to the necessary placements and services. A school cannot escape their legal obligation to provide a free, appropriate public education to every child by simply saying they do not have special education services as long as the school receives some federal funding.

Most school districts are prepared for situations when a child's special needs cannot be met by the school. For large school districts in highly populated cities, the provision of services and placement is usually not a problem. If your child's school does not have the appropriate classroom placement or services, the correct setting likely exists in a nearby school, to which your child will be provided transportation. If you child has needs for special services that are not ordinarily provided by her school, the district may bring in a specialist to your child's campus. In smaller areas, two or three school districts will often work together to share resources.

If your child's school district refuses to provide necessary placement or services by claiming it does not have what your child needs, it is in violation of the law. Parents in this situation are best advised to consult with an advocate or lawyer.

What if my child goes to a private school?

Children with disabilities who are in a private school by parental choice still have rights and access to special education under IDEA 2004. Procedures for evaluation and services are the same as for children enrolled in the local public school. The privately schooled child is entitled to a services plan that describes the specific special education and related services the school district will provide. The services plan is similar to an IEP. A representative from the private school must provide input or attend the services plan meeting. There is a formula in IDEA 2004 about how much money the public school district must spend on disabled children in private schools. Often this service is limited to consultation with the private school.

Services provided to the disabled child may be at the private school's expense, but are not required to take place there. If services are provided off-site from the private school, the school district must supply necessary transportation. Transportation is only required from the private school to the location of the special education service, not from home to the private school.

Even though services are available for AD children in private school, it is usually not the best solution. These children typically function better in a school designed solely for AD children or in a public school with services for the AD child.

Will special education stigmatize my child?

When parents think of special education, they usually reflect back to unpleasant childhood memories of special education students at their school. Children with disabilities were kept completely isolated from the general education students and were not allowed to share recess and lunch periods or participate in general PE classes, and were prevented from attending school social activities.

Fortunately, special education has come a long way since then. Children are included in the general education setting to the greatest extent possible and are no longer segregated. Still, parents worry about their child's self-esteem if they are labeled as a special-needs child. This worry usually lives more in the imaginations of the parents than in the self-image of the child. When parents come to understand that labeling a child as a special education student is a necessary entry procedure to obtaining services, they are able to decrease their fears.

General education and special education teachers are aware of the teasing that special education students may receive from their nondisabled peers and typically work to teach all students that special education is not negative and is just a different way for students to learn. Parents can reinforce this with their emotional support of their child.

What should I know about my child's special education records?

Schools are required by federal and state laws to maintain certain records and to have them available to you upon request. The federal law Family Educational Rights and Privacy Act (FERPA) establishes minimum requirements for maintaining, protecting, and providing access to school records. State laws may have additional protections.

Under FERPA, parents have a right to all files and documents maintained by the school system that contain information related to their child. This includes any documents that identify your child by name, social security number, school identification number, or other data that make the records traceable back to your child.

Your child's records will be broken into several files. The cumulative file includes personal identification, academic achievement test scores, teacher reports, and report cards. The confidential file holds written reports from the school's evaluations, any evaluation reports and records you provided, IEPs, written documents between yourself and school personnel, and reports from IEP team members.

Some schools will keep a compliance file that holds documents that demonstrate the school's compliance with IDEA 2004. This would include reports of eligibility meetings and correspondence between the school and parents. Finally, some schools keep a discipline file where they hold records regarding suspensions and expulsion.

Who can access my child's records?

Special education records are quite secure, and there is little need to worry about negative consequences from having a special education file.

All documents related to special education are permanently kept in a file separate from your child's usual academic records. These files are marked confidential and are accessible only by school personnel who have a need to know. Special education teachers, school counselors, and any specialist providing special education services to your child are considered as having a need to know. Teachers who will not be addressing your child's special education needs have no cause to read your child's confidential file.

Only parents or guardians have the legal authority to allow the release of their child's school records, including the confidential file. Once the child turns eighteen, the authority transfers to him. When the parents or adult child request the school records to be released, only the general education file is sent. Only with specific written request can the confidential file be released.

Parents and the senior high school student will want to consider releasing the most recent IEP to the student's college of choice. Colleges provide 504 accommodations that may assist your child in her college education.

What are the exceptions to the privacy of my child's records?

The federal laws of FERPA and IDEA 2004 protect your child's records from being shown to anyone without your written consent. However, as with all records, there are always exceptions. The law allows for access to your child's school record by the following individuals or agencies:

- School officials with a legitimate educational interest
- School officials in the district to which your child intends to transfer
- Certain state and national education agencies for purposes of enforcing federal laws
- Anyone to whom a state statute requires the school to report information to
- Accrediting and research organizations helping the school, provided they guarantee confidentiality
- Student financial aid officials

- People who have court orders, provided the school makes reasonable efforts to notify the parents prior to releasing the records
- Law enforcement and judicial authorities in certain cases

What most parents are concerned about are potential colleges and employers gaining access to the confidential file. Unless specifically authorized in writing to do so, the school district may not release the confidential file to a college or employer.

How can I find out how my child is doing in the classroom?

In the absence of a note sent home from the teacher, parents assume things are going well. Come report card time, parents are often unpleasantly surprised.

While some teachers will make frequent contact through notes or phone calls to parents, unfortunately the majority are simply too busy to do so. Unless teachers are asked to report progress, many wait until report card time, far too late, to inform parents about their AD child.

If your child has a written IEP or a Section 504 accommodation plan, request that the method and frequency of contact between yourself and the teacher be written into the plan. The teacher must comply with what is written in either plan, regardless of how busy he is.

Rather than wait for the teacher to make contact, parents of AD children should contact the teacher early in the school year and ask what method he would prefer to keep you informed about your child's schoolwork and behavior. Have a plan in mind that would be easy for the teacher to use. Email, voice mail, or a behavior chart can be quick methods that will not burden the teacher's time.

Should my child repeat a grade to give him time to mature?

Children with AD are emotionally and socially delayed at a minimum of three years. Behaviors their peers have outgrown persist in AD children well beyond what is expected. This immaturity may lead parents to consider having their child repeat a grade in order to give him time to catch up to his classmates. This may sound good in theory, but in reality, it does not work and is not supported by research.

Holding a child back for a year might work if he were evenly delayed one year in all areas. However, AD children have very scattered emotional development. A child may have the vocabulary of adult, the frustration tolerance of a three-year-old, and the social skills of a second-grade student. Given the large gaps in emotional maturity, there is no one grade level that will even the playing field for the AD child.

Children do not catch up or outgrow their symptoms throughout their childhood, much less in one school year. Holding an AD child back one year fails to bring about emotional growth. The best solution is to seek an IEP or Section 504.

How are behavior problems handled through special education?

Teachers generally try to motivate children to perform well and cooperate with classroom rules with the use of praise, encouragement, and privileges. For many children with AD, these behavioral techniques are insufficient and the child is often found to disrupt the teacher and classmates. For such children, either the parent or teacher may request the assistance of a behaviorist to perform a behavioral functional assessment.

In this special type of assessment, a behaviorist will observe your child in the classroom, looking for when the problem behavior arises, what triggers it, what consequences are used, and how effective the consequences are. The behaviorist is looking for underlying causes of the problem behavior to determine if it can be prevented.

If the behaviorist determines that a behavior-modification program is likely to be successful in decreasing or eliminating the behavior, she will design a plan. The goal is to modify the behavior so that the child will be able to remain in the general education classroom. The behaviorist will train the teacher how to implement the plan. The plan will generally involve one or more specific behaviors with methods to prevent them, rewards to give, and methods to keep track of success.

How are suspensions and expulsions handled for special education students?

Children with AD are more likely to get suspended or expelled from school than their nondisabled peers. Under IDEA 2004, there are specific rules regarding suspensions and expulsions for special education students that protect them from excessive and unproductive disciplinary action. Suspensions of more than ten consecutive days require certain actions on the part of the school district. IDEA 2004 has made major changes in how discipline is handled for disabled students. It is best to consult an advocate or a special education lawyer who specializes in discipline issues if the school is threatening expulsion or change of placement caused by a discipline issue. Under Section 504, the child is not given the same protection. The school does not have to keep the child in school while they perform an assessment for the offending behavior.

Chapter 10

IMPROVING BEHAVIOR

- Why is parent education important?
- What should I tell the adults in my child's life about his Asperger's Disorder?
- Should I work on changing my child's behavior or just accept him the way he is?
- What are the stresses faced by children and teens with Asperger's Disorder?
- What behavior problems are my child likely to have?
- What is behavior modification?
- What are the ABC's of behavior modification?
- What is positive reinforcement?
- How can I use positive reinforcement to improve my child's behavior?
- What are the other behavior-modification methods?
- How can I use reinforcement and punishment to improve my child's behavior?
- What is shaping?
- How can I use shaping to improve my child's behavior?
- What is backward chaining?
- What is extinction?
- How can I use extinction to improve my child's behavior?
- What is Functional Analysis of Behavior?
- How does Functional Analysis of Behavior help to improve my child's behavior?
- How do I create a Functional Analysis of Behavior for my child?
- What challenges should I expect when using behavior modification?
- How important is consistency when using behavior modification?
- How can I use behavior modification to help my child do his daily tasks?
- What is the best way to correct my child's misbehavior?
- Should I try to reason with my child when he is upset?
- How can I best help my child when he is having an outburst?
- Should I allow my child to give himself a time-out?
- What behaviors should I insist my child do?
- What are predictable consequences?
- Nothing I do makes any difference—now what?

Why is parent education important?

Learning that your child has AD probably comes as a mix of upset and relief. It is certainly upsetting to learn that your child has a disorder, but at the same time many parents feel relieved to finally have a name to put to the problems they have observed in their child for years. It is important that you give yourself permission to feel sad and disappointed and to grieve the loss of the dreams you had. It is normal to feel these emotions and healthy to acknowledge and talk about them.

Once you let the grieving happen, you are emotionally free to spend your energies learning all you can about AD. With knowledge and understanding comes the compassion that your child needs. The more you understand the disorder the better job you will do in knowing which behaviors to tolerate, which to discipline, which to push, and which to just give up on. You will be better able to assist your child's teachers in how to best teach him and better able to explain to friends, relatives, and coaches about why your child behaves the way he does.

What should I tell the adults in my child's life about his Asperger's Disorder?

Because AD is a newly recognized disorder, your disclosure of your child's AD may be the first time that adults in your child's life have heard of it. Few teachers will have had much training and experience. The more the adults in your child's life understand AD the better job they will do supporting your child. Without knowledge of AD, it is very easy for any adult to unknowingly misjudge your child as uncooperative and disrespectful.

Adults in your child's life may suddenly feel nervous, believing they are not skilled enough to help your child. You can decrease their fears by telling them that one of the most important skills they can provide takes no actual training, only unconditional positive regard. An adult who is kind, patient, complimentary, and protective will go a long way in not only making your child feel worthwhile but also in modeling for others how to treat her with kindness. An adult who shows irritability and impatience and makes critical remarks to or about your child is likely to cause others to do the same.

Provide your child's grandparents, aunts and uncles, neighbors, baby-sitters, coaches, teachers, and siblings with information about AD. Loan or buy them a copy of this book.

Should I work on changing my child's behavior or just accept him the way he is?

You are in good company if you struggle with trying to get others to accept your child the way he is and getting him to try to adapt to the world. It is exhausting to think about having to work on the numerous symptoms your child displays. It can be easy to convince yourself that some of them are just not important and the world should learn to be more tolerant of those with differences. You may think, *So what if he can't get along on the playground? If he can't play cooperatively, he can always play alone.* If you adopt this approach, you can expect him to spend the rest of his life alone, having no friends.

Each behavior by itself may be easy to accept, but the overall picture must be kept in mind. Imagine what his life will be like if he does not adapt to the world he lives in. Ignoring his deficits will have lifelong implications. If you fail to provide him with the tools to get along in life, you are boxing him in for life. If he is not pushed to learn skills and adapt, he will be forced to live a restricted and rigid life without choices.

What are the stresses faced by children and teens with Asperger's Disorder?

School is probably your child's greatest challenge, source of stress, and cause of behavior problems. The classroom can be overwhelming. In the midst of trying to learn, his mind may be filled with the stress of the visual and auditory stimulation, obsessing about his special interest, feeling embarrassed about the teasing he endured during recess, frustrated that he cannot ask every question he wants, intolerant of what he views as his peers' ignorance on his topic of interest, upset at the change in the schedule, bored with the lesson, and too humiliated to admit that he does not understand what the teacher is saying. Imagine all this being your normal life, occurring day after day. Now add having to do homework, cooperate with parents, get along with siblings, and try to make friends.

The buildup of the stress from trying to cope with the various events, tasks, and challenges of the day is often the cause of what seems to be an unprovoked outburst.

It is a wonder that AD children do not have more behavior problems. Understanding his disorder and the difficulty it presents at every moment of the day makes it easier to be compassionate when he has behavior problems.

What behavior problems are my child likely to have?

Having AD does not necessarily mean your child is going to have significant behavior problems. The likelihood of significant behavior problems increases dramatically if your child has a coexisting behavior disorder such as ADD, ADHD, or ODD.

By itself AD is not a behavior disorder and, with good management techniques to address the symptoms, your child may experience only mild to moderate behavior problems. The behavioral problems that children and teens with AD do display can often be traced to their inability to cope with the symptoms of the disorder. Unfortunately, AD children and teens are not good at identifying or verbalizing what is upsetting them, and it can be quite difficult for you as a parent to figure it out. Techniques in this chapter will help you discover causes and learn techniques to manage these problems:

- Noncompliance
- Tantrums
- Anger outbursts
- Aggression
- Procrastination
- Screaming
- Yelling
- Refusal

What is behavior modification?

Behavior modification is considered equal in importance to social skills therapy in helping children and teens with AD. This type of therapy, while its goals are to help your child, can only be done with your active involvement. You become the behavior modifier at home, essentially serving in the role of a behavior therapist.

While behavior modification is relatively easy to learn, the challenge comes in finding the motivation to use it on a consistent basis. Research clearly documents that when the skills are used predictably and reliably, substantial improvements are seen, both in the child's behavior and in the parent-child relationship. When parents are inconsistent or stop using the techniques, their child's behavior deteriorates to the pre-behavior-modification level. The frustration for many parents is that they have to use behavior modification seven days a week, 365 days a year, year after year. If they slack off, their child's behavior deteriorates.

There are a variety of behavior-modification techniques you will learn in this chapter, including:

- Positive Reinforcement
- Positive Punishment
- Negative Punishment
- Negative Reinforcement
- Shaping
- Backward Chaining
- Extinction
- Applied Behavioral Analysis
- Functional Behavioral Analysis
- Floor Time

What are the ABC's of behavior modification?

Based on the belief that behavior occurs for a reason, behavior modification seeks to look at what causes behaviors and what encourages or discourages them.

Antecedents are the events that happen just prior to a behavior. Antecedents can increase or decrease the chance that a behavior occurs. If your child packs her backpack when you remind her, the antecedent of your reminder is effective. If your son tantrums when you tell him to turn off his computer, the antecedent of telling him to turn it off is not effective.

Behaviors are the actions that follow immediately after the antecedents. Packing the backpack, turning off the computer, and throwing a tantrum are behaviors.

Consequences are what happen immediately after the behavior. In behavior-modification language, "consequence" does not mean a punishment or something negative. Consequences are simply the results of a behavior and can be good, bad, or neutral. Consequences might include allowing your daughter to watch television once she has packed her backpack or giving in to your son's tantrum and letting him have more time on the computer. If the consequence is favorable the behavior will likely repeat. If it is unfavorable it is less likely to repeat.

What is positive reinforcement?

Undoubtedly the most commonly used behavior modification technique, positive reinforcement is the giving of something pleasurable in anticipation that it will improve behavior. You probably are already an expert at positive reinforcement; each time you praise your child you are using positive reinforcement in hopes that he will repeat the desired behavior.

What you give in positive reinforcement is called a reinforcer. There are an infinite number of possible reinforcers. In order for the reinforcer to be effective in increasing desirable behavior, it must be something your child likes. If you give him a lima bean when he completes his homework, chances are he will not do much homework tomorrow. However, if you give him a hug, pat, smile, time with television, computer or video games, a food treat, or points toward a prize, he will be more likely to do his homework the next day.

Positive reinforcement can also increase undesirable behaviors. If you give your child a cookie each time she tantrums, you are increasing the chance that she will tantrum in order to earn a cookie. Understanding that *positive* means giving and *reinforcement* means increasing, you can use positive reinforcement to give things to increase desirable behaviors and avoid giving things that increase undesirable behavior.

How can I use positive reinforcement to improve my child's behavior?

Positive reinforcement is a very effective behavioral technique for increasing appropriate behavior. Praise is the easiest and most commonly used positive reinforcer. Being overly sensitive to criticism, AD children are hungry for and responsive to praise. However, unlike most children, who are happy to be told their behavior is good, AD children seem to prefer praise for their intellectual choices. Rather than telling your child, "You are doing a good job on your homework," you can appeal to his craving for admiration of his intelligence by calling attention to his wise choices: "That was a smart decision to get going on your homework so you have plenty of time to work on your rock collection tonight." Look for opportunities to praise your child. He has so many opportunities for others to point out his wrongdoings—he needs you to point out what he does right.

Positive reinforcement can also be used in the form of a behavior chart where your child earns a point for every task he is expected to perform. He can trade his points for food treats, privileges, or items. Don't worry if he wants to spend most of his points on engaging in or purchasing items for his special interest.

What are the other behavior-modification methods?

Three other methods of changing your child's behavior include positive punishment, negative punishment, and negative reinforcement.

Positive punishment is the giving of something in order to decrease an undesirable behavior. A spanking is a form of positive punishment. Even though a spanking is actually a very negative experience, in behavior modification language, *positive* always means giving. *Punishment* means it is designed to decrease a behavior. Yelling at your child when you catch him playing with matches decreases the chance he will play with matches again.

Negative punishment is when you take away something in order to decrease a behavior. Taking away your child's computer in order to get him to stop lying about his homework is an example of negative punishment. *Negative* in behavior-modification language means to remove something. *Punishment* here again means to decrease the unwanted behavior. Taking away the car keys when your son fails three classes is negative punishment. You are hoping to decrease his failing grades by doing this.

Negative reinforcement increases behavior because you take something unpleasant away. We have all been trained through negative reinforcement to put on our seat belts in order to stop the buzz our car makes until we have done so. You raise your voice and lecture your daughter about not cleaning her room. She gets up from her video game and begins to clean her room and you therefore stop the lecture. She learns that in order to stop you from yelling in the future, she must clean her room.

Anything you do that *increases* your child's behavior is called *reinforcement* and any anything you do that *decreases* behavior is called *punishment*. If you *present* something after the behavior it is called *positive*, and if you *remove* something it is called *negative*.

The entire foundation of behavior modification is based upon these four forms of intervention and thus you should work to understand them fully. This chart can help make it simpler to determine the methods and goals of each of these techniques.

	Reinforcement—to increase	Punishment—to decrease
Positive—Giving	Increase Behavior	Decrease Behavior
Negative—Taking Away	Increase Behavior	Decrease Behavior

How can I use reinforcement and punishment to improve my child's behavior?

Make a list of all the behaviors you want your child to do. Next to each one, write down whether you want the behavior to increase or decrease. Write which behavior-modification technique you will use for each behavior. For behaviors you want to increase, you will want to use positive reinforcement or negative reinforcement.

For behaviors you want to decrease, you will want to use positive punishment or negative punishment.

Behavior	Goal	Technique	Consequence
Starts home-work at 4 p.m.	Increase	Positive reinforcement	Praise, 5 points
Turns off TV when told	Increase	Negative reinforcement	Raise voice until TV off
Breaks curfew	Decrease	Negative punishment	Lose car for 1 week
Jumps on furniture	Decrease	Positive punishment	Raise voice to stop
Brushes teeth	Increase	Positive reinforcement	Praise, read story

Since we know that children and teens respond better to positive reinforcement, you should try to use this tool as often as possible. Behaviors you want to decrease can be viewed in the opposite direction. For example, you want your teenage son to stop breaking curfew and you use negative punishment of removing his car privileges for one week. Knowing that punishment may work less effectively than positive reinforcement, you can change the behavior to "Come home by curfew" with the goal of increasing this behavior. Using positive reinforcement, you can reward your child with a tank of gas, or a later curfew, or spending money, thereby increasing his motivation to come home by curfew. If this fails to result in him making curfew, then negative punishment of removing the car just might.

Behavior	Goal	Technique	Consequence
Home by curfew	Increase	Positive reinforcement	Mom buys tank of gas

What is shaping?

Shaping involves the use of positive reinforcement to teach a desired behavior. A desired behavior is broken down into baby steps and your child is taught one step at a time. You praise and/or reward him for his attempts and his small successes towards the behavior. Shaping uses only positive reinforcement. No negative reinforcement or punishment is used.

Keep expectations small until step one is achieved. Praise effort as well as success. When step one is mastered, step two is taught and reinforced until success is consistently achieved. The third step is added, then the fourth, etc., until the entire behavior is achieved. Once your child can do the entire behavior, he is prompted each step of the way as he performs the behavior. As he demonstrates consistent success in the behavior, your prompts are given less often in a process called fading. Eventually your child will be able to do the entire behavior with only a prompt to start it.

If the behavior needs to take place in more than one setting, once your child has mastered the skill in one setting, he is then asked to perform the behavior in a second setting, a process called generalization.

How can I use shaping to improve my child's behavior?

Much of what you do to help your child learn skills and improve her behavior uses shaping. Make a list of the tasks, chores, and behaviors that you expect of your child. Mark those that he struggles with, break them down into tiny steps, and write a step-by-step procedure. These written steps are for your use to guide you in shaping your child's behavior, not for him to see. Decrease your expectations and set goals for your child to achieve only step one of each of the challenging behaviors. Take joy both when he tries and when he succeeds and share your happiness with him. Continue on with a very enthusiastic shaping program that progresses slowly and adds minor increases in expectations only after sure success in the prior step. You can use shaping on any behavior.

You may feel some frustration that your child is not learning the skill fast enough. This is most likely to occur in more challenging behaviors such as doing homework independently. Be careful not to add steps too fast. Unless your child automatically starts to do the next step, let him experience a few weeks of success before you add the next step.

What is backward chaining?

Backward chaining is very similar to shaping. It involves the same method of teaching a behavior, except that the behavior is taught in a reverse order. Instead of teaching the task from the beginning, you do the entire task with the exception of the very last step, which you save for him to do. Positive reinforcement is used for attempts and success. Once he has the last step of the task mastered, you add the second-to-last step, and so on. The backward approach can be more effective in situations that seem overwhelming to your child. He may view the unmade bed as an impossible task and may do whatever it takes to avoid having to make it. If he instead sees the entire bed made and he only has to put his stuffed animals on top, the task appears far less daunting. Once he has consistently been able to put the stuffed animals on the bed, you can add the step of pulling the spread over the pillow until he has mastered this with ease and without conflict. Pulling the spread up over the bed is added next, and so on until eventually he can make the entire bed.

What is extinction?

Extinction is designed to decrease undesirable behavior. It involves the purposeful and persistent ignoring of unwanted behavior. Your strengths in ignoring must be stronger and outlast the strength of your child's negative behavior. Sometimes extinction is easy to do, such as when you ignore your child's interrupting you while you are talking. You keep talking and do not look at him, touch him, or acknowledge him in any way. The hope is that if he gets absolutely nothing from you, he will figure out that persisting is useless and he better find another way to get your attention.

Extinction during tantrums is more challenging. Many AD children have far more stamina in their tantrums than their parents have in extinction. If extinction is to be effective, you must stay firm in your ignoring. This means no words, no touching, no gestures, and no eye contact. Unless your child is in danger, you ignore him until he stops the tantrum and begins to engage in appropriate behavior. The instant he uses nice words, apologizes, or begins to comply with your original request, you give him positive reinforcement. The idea is for him to learn that he gets absolutely nothing for inappropriate behavior, but gets positive attention for appropriate behavior.

How can I use extinction to improve my child's behavior?

Extinction can be used to decrease and eventually eliminate undesirable behaviors. Some behaviors are responsive to extinction while others are not. In order to decide if extinction might work, you must determine if your attention is part of what your child wants. Crying, whining, tugging, interrupting, throwing tantrums, yelling, throwing, hitting, and holding his breath are behaviors that usually are motivated at least in part by a child's desire for his parents' attention.

Other behaviors, however, are rewarding enough to the child that they do not need your attention. Jumping on furniture, sneaking food treats, and annoying a sibling are behaviors that are usually pleasant all by themselves and will actually increase with extinction.

Behaviors that you choose to use extinction for must be safe for your child and others. As long as he cannot truly hurt himself with his behavior, you can use extinction. Be sure that you are in a situation where you can use extinction and will not have to give in to your child's behavior because he is bothering others or embarrassing you.

What is Functional Analysis of Behavior?

Functional Analysis of Behavior (FAB) or Applied Behavior Analysis (ABA) is a process with the goal of determining why a particular behavior occurs. Instead of simply making a plan to stop a behavior, FAB is based upon the belief that behaviors occur for specific reasons and the fastest way to stop an unwanted behavior is to find out why it happens.

You can begin FAB by first selecting a behavior to decrease. Keep notes that carefully describe the unwanted behavior in specific terms so that an outsider would be able to recognize it easily. The unwanted behavior is referred to as the target behavior. Once the target behavior is clearly defined, spend at least one week making notes that include:

- Location—where the target behavior occurs
- Intensity—how severe the target behavior is
- Frequency—how often the target behavior occurs
- Duration—how long the target behavior lasts
- Antecedents—what events occur just before the target behavior starts
- Consequences—what events happen as a result of the target behavior
- Course—how the target behavior is displayed; if any changes occur before it stops

How does Functional Analysis of Behavior help to improve my child's behavior?

The analysis described above usually reveals a pattern of the behavior. You should be able to tell from your notes why the inappropriate behavior is occurring. The next step is to find an alternative acceptable behavior. After this you can design a plan that will allow your child to stop the inappropriate behavior and start the desirable behavior in its place.

Such a plan involves:

- Preventing the antecedents—stopping the cause
- Changing the consequence—making sure the consequence is not rewarding
- Modifying the environment—changing the environment to prevent the behavior
- Teaching appropriate behavior—demonstrating/role playing appropriate behavior
- Prompting appropriate behavior—reminders to do the appropriate behavior
- Rewarding appropriate behavior—giving praise, rewards, and privileges for appropriate behavior

Once the plan is put into place, records are kept to monitor the target behavior to see if your plan is working to decrease the undesirable behavior. Expect your plan to need several modifications as you use it over the course of several weeks. Through the process of trial and error and your detailed record keeping, it should be relatively easy to tell what is working and what needs to be changed.

How do I create a Functional Analysis of Behavior for my child?

Let's say your child becomes upset in the car whenever you are driving him and his brother somewhere. Both boys fight, but it seems that your son with AD is the one who starts it. You have to figure out what starts it and what you can do to change it.

Your FAB might look something like this:

Behavior	Yelling, screaming, hitting brother
Location	In the car when his brother is with him
Intensity	6 on a scale of 1–10
Frequency	Every time brother is in car, usually 5 days a week, on school days
Duration	Lasts entire drive home, about 20 minutes
Antecedents	His brother sings and hums loudly
Consequences	I yell at him to leave his brother alone and accept that his brother has a right to sing and hum even if he does not like it
Course	He escalates every few minutes and does not calm down until we get home and he goes to his room
Preventing the antecedents	Brother is told to not sing or hum when others are in the car
Changing the consequence	I prompt his brother about the new rule to not sing or hum when others are in the car
Modifying the environment	I have both boys' CD players and headsets in their seats to listen to
Teaching appropriate behavior	I teach him how to distract himself from what annoys him, teach relaxation skills, and how to use his words with his brother
Prompting appropriate behavior	I remind him what choices he has for appropriate behavior. I can do this as soon as we get in the car.
Rewarding appropriate behavior	He can get a snack when we get home if he does not yell, scream, or hit. He can earn bonus points if he uses his coping skills of words, relaxation, or distraction.

What challenges should I expect when using behavior modification?

Behavior modification can present many challenges with your AD child or teen. You may have to purposely look for behaviors to praise. Finding items and activities to use for positive reinforcement can be difficult as your child may have few things that he is excited to earn. On the other hand, his special interest may be so fulfilling that all he wants is a chance to read his book on trains or earn one more coin for his penny collection.

Certain behaviors unique to the AD child and teen are highly resistant to extinction. Using extinction to ignore a child's incessant talking and repeated questioning may be futile as those with AD find talking so rewarding that they do not need you to participate and they won't really notice if you are not listening. The other challenge with extinction is that when you begin to use this technique, your child will more than likely increase his inappropriate behavior even more than before. Your initial impression that extinction is not working is premature. An extinction burst is the expected increase seen immediately after extinction is implemented. If you can stand your ground and keep using the technique, your child will decrease his inappropriate behavior.

How important is consistency when using behavior modification?

Regardless of age or disorder, behavior modification for any reason requires consistency. If you quit using behavior modification, your child usually quits behaving appropriately.

Consistency is important for all children, but even more critical for children and teens with AD. These children like things to be highly predictable so they know exactly what will happen and when it will happen. Routine helps your child feel less anxious, which in turn will translate into improved behavior as he will not be having outbursts or defiance in reaction to unpredictability.

This all works to your advantage as your child will function at his best with a highly structured, predictable, and consistent life at home. Behavior modification helps you to create clearly defined rules, consequences, and schedules. If you forget to give your child his reinforcer, chances are he will remind you until you give it to him.

True, it is hard to be consistent. No doubt about it, all the things parents have to do to raise a child with AD are exhausting. Try to not let yourself be so overwhelmed that you are just too tired to be consistent.

How can I use behavior modification to help my child to do his daily tasks?

Children with AD can often become irritable when told what to do and prefer to have a sense of control over their tasks. You and your child can make task cards with each card having a picture and/or a short description of the task on one side and a step-by-step list on the other side.

Give a younger child one card and tell him that when he is done with the task he is to bring the card back to you. Praise him when he returns the card and give him the next one. Older children can tack the cards on a low-hanging bulletin board in the order they are to be completed. Older children may use a small file box where the cards are numbered and placed in order.

The cards eliminate telling him what to do by nagging and reminding. Cards work better than a list, as your child only has to think about the one behavior on the card. The picture gives a visual cue, which for many AD children is easier than listening or reading. For those that read, the list on the back tells them what to do step-by-step.

What is the best way to correct my child's misbehavior?

AD children are particularly sensitive to criticism. Quick to dole it out, they will avoid being embarrassed at all costs. They will not admit they are wrong. They will not say they do not know an answer or that they do not understand something. They are reluctant to ask for help, say they were not paying attention, or that they forgot what they are supposed to be doing. Even the kindest of parents can inadvertently spark an outburst when correcting misbehavior. Some tips for parents include:

- Avoid using critical words
- Matter-of-factly describe the misbehavior
- Offer a better choice for behavior
- Gently teach the impact on others of misbehavior
- Avoid pointing out misbehavior in front of others
- Create a secret signal you can use to prompt the child to assess his own behavior
- Ask your child if help is needed by whispering quietly so others do not hear
- Create a secret signal the child can use to let you know he needs your help
- Do not ask the child to admit wrongdoing
- Keep all discussions about the child's misbehavior private

Should I try to reason with my child when he is upset?

When children with AD become upset, they become more rigid in their thinking and "get stuck" with a thought. It can be difficult to interrupt their thought patterns and get them to see an alternative viewpoint. While it seems rational to try to reason and calmly explain the situation and persuade your child to find an alternative thought and behavior, her mind gets stuck on a thought, and like a needle stuck in a record, cannot switch gears. If you persist in trying to change his thought and behavior, you can often precipitate a meltdown.

Most people do not think clearly when they are upset, but those with AD have far greater trouble with this than most. It is as if they have two minds and when the emotional mind is in full gear the rational mind shuts off. A more helpful approach is to stop in your tracks and change the subject, redirect your child to an alternative pleasant activity, ask her to perform a particular duty she likes, or simply stop talking or leave the room. You can revisit the topic later when your child is calm and can hear what you have to say.

How can I best help my child when he is having an outburst?

AD children and teens are sure to have outbursts, so it is best to try to prevent them, prepare for when they do occur, and de-escalate them as quickly as possible. AD children and teens need to be taught how to tell if they are getting upset and how to rate the severity. A drawing of a thermometer with words and/or faces can be used to help your child learn to recognize and verbalize his upset on a scale from irritation to outrage. Cool down methods can be written or drawn next to each stage of upset to describe how to calm down, such as taking three deep breaths for minor irritation, squeezing and relaxing hands when angry, and going to his safe place when enraged.

Some tips that can help your child when he is upset include:

- Remain calm regardless of how out-of-control he gets
- Prompt him to use his cool down methods
- Be alert to small signs of emotional upset and prompt for ways to resolve it
- Attempt to redirect an impending outburst by distracting with a pleasurable task
- Praise his attempts at cooling down
- Praise him when he brings himself under control
- Let him pick someone he can call or go to when he feels the need
- Provide a safe place to go to when he feels as if he going to explode
- Stay out of power struggles
- Realize something caused the tantrum even if you can't tell what
- Accept that you cannot stop a tantrum
- Realize she cannot control herself right at this moment
- Save the talk for later when she is calm
- Keep quiet—he can't listen in the midst of a tantrum and it will only escalate it
- Be a soothing presence
- Prevent situations you know cause tantrums
- Focus on right now; forget about the fifty-nine other times he threw a tantrum
- Let him have the time and space to have a meltdown and regain self-control
- Do not issue any demands other than for safety needs during an outburst

Should I allow my child to give himself a time-out?

Serious outbursts can be prevented by creating a place for your child to give himself a time-out. This type of time-out is different from those used for misbehavior. This is a place for retreat, not punishment. You can help him create his own safe haven in the house or yard. Let him put things in his safe place that he feels would help soothe him. He may want a beanbag to sit in, pillows to lie on, a favorite stuffed animal to hug, or a small ball to squeeze. While time-out is a common term, you and your child may want to create a more positive name. He will make more use of his time-out place if he helps select a secret signal for you and him to use to let one another know when a break is needed. The location must be safe and prevent harm to himself, others, and property. The break should last as long as your child needs to calm himself down. Expect that initially he may "abuse" the privilege by taking more breaks than are really necessary. Don't worry about this, as it simply gives him more practice recognizing his stress signals, responding appropriately by removing himself and going to a safe place to calm down. The number of breaks will diminish when the novelty wears off and he learns that he is not able to avoid cooperation with requests, chores, and tasks by taking a time-out.

What behaviors should I insist my child do?

Each parent has certain behaviors they will not tolerate as well as ones they are not concerned with. Some parents will not tolerate talking back while others cannot accept a messy room. Because AD children engage in so many inappropriate behaviors, it is impossible to set a consequence for them all. Even if you tried, you would be unable to point out to your child each of his misbehaviors. Sometimes your child will be simultaneously engaging in so many inappropriate actions that you won't know which one to tell him to stop.

Instead, you must determine which behaviors and tasks *you* believe are the most important. You have to choose your battles. It is easier to first make a list of which behaviors and tasks you can let go. A clean room should be on the top of the list of behaviors to give up.

Topping the list of behaviors that all children should do include brushing teeth, bathing, going to school, and doing some homework. Behaviors that all children should be disciplined for include physical violence, property destruction, cursing, and threats of violence.

What are predictable consequences?

It is a daunting prospect to attempt to create a consequence for all the problem behaviors your AD child engages in. Even if you could write a rule for every misdeed, it's unrealistic to think that you would have the time, patience, and stamina to develop consequences for each one. Fortunately, by using predictable consequences, you don't have to.

Predictable consequences are the automatic results of behavior that occur without you having to do anything. If your son refuses to wear his jacket to school, he will be cold. If he throws his toy in anger and breaks it, he no longer has the pleasure of that toy. These are situations where the punishment simply presents itself. Parents do not have to be the punisher in situations that have a predictable consequence. Instead they can be empathic parents who calmly say, "That's what happens, honey, when you don't take an umbrella—you get rained on." Nature doled out the punishment and you can save your discipline for situations when there is not a predictable consequence.

Nothing I do makes any difference—now what?

This feeling is more common than not in parents of AD children. No matter what you try, nothing seems to make any lasting difference. There is a good reason for this.

Nothing you do as a parent will cure the disorder. The behaviors that your AD child exhibits will be with him throughout his childhood and adolescence. You can help him to manage the symptoms but you will not eliminate them. You will be far less frustrated if you understand that parenting techniques are designed to *manage* the symptoms of AD by decreasing their frequency, intensity, and severity, not cure them.

AD children are not your average children and they do not readily respond to the usual parenting methods. If life is not more manageable after you have learned the behavior-modification techniques and have consistently used them in your home, then it is time to seek assistance. A child psychologist can work with you to teach you where changes need to be made. Once life is stable at home, periodic visits to the psychologist can help keep your parenting in sync with your child's changes and development.

Chapter 11

SELF-ESTEEM

- Does AD affect self-esteem?
- How much self-esteem do children with Asperger's Disorder have?
- How can I tell if my child has low self-esteem?
- Can a child have too much self-esteem?
- How will special education affect my child's self-esteem?
- How can my child's teacher help with self-esteem?
- How does teasing affect self-esteem?
- How can I help my child cope with being teased?
- Can extracurricular activities increase self-esteem?
- Can praise increase self-esteem?
- How can compliments increase my child's self-esteem?
- How does my parenting style affect my child's self-esteem?
- How can unconditional love help with self-esteem?
- Can helping others increase my child's self-esteem?
- How can I help my child stop negative self-talk?
- How can I help my child accept his weaknesses?
- How do I give my child a realistic sense of self?
- How do I help my child find a sense of competence?
- How can Snapshots enhance my child's self-esteem?
- What can I do to improve my child's self-esteem?

Does AD affect self-esteem?

Having any type of psychological disorder can have a negative effect on self-esteem. AD is far more vulnerable than other disorders. Most other disorders in children are not so easily seen by other people. As long as others do not know he has a disorder, the child can avoid embarrassment. AD, on the other hand, cannot be hidden. The overt social problems displayed by the AD child are frequently responded to with negative comments from others. Both the inability to hide the disorder and the negative feedback he receives contribute to feelings of low self-worth.

Further contributing to negative self-esteem is that unlike other disorders, AD does not elicit sympathy. While a depressed child might be treated with more kindness and patience, and never told, "Stop being depressed," the AD child engenders frustration and impatience. Being told repeatedly to stop talking, stop interrupting, or talk about something else for a change leads the AD child to feel as if he is always doing something wrong. This of course leads to lower self-esteem.

Having AD is strongly associated with depression in adolescent and adult years.

How much self-esteem do children with Asperger's Disorder have?

Self-esteem is not a black-and-white situation of having or not having it. Nor is it something that can really be measured. Rather it is on a continuum from low to high. Unfortunately, having AD is almost a guarantee of being on the low end of self-worth. AD children often have low self-esteem regarding the main categories of school, family, and friends.

As AD children move into their teen years, their self-esteem is generally quite low and their risk for depression increases. They clearly see that they do not measure up to their peers in terms of being socially accepted. Unless effective treatment is sought, this pattern continues to become more severe as they move into later adolescence and adulthood.

Fortunately children do not have just one self-esteem. You can help your child develop multiple self-esteems. The more activities and experiences he has where he feels good about himself, the higher his overall level of self-esteem is going to be. Self-esteem can be found in simple experiences. As many AD children shy away from new experiences, particularly those that involve the potential for failure or social rejection, be sure to create simple experiences that offer a high chance of success.

How can I tell if my child has low self-esteem?

Children with low self-esteem will reveal it through their words. Listen to what your child says about himself. Children with low self-esteem talk negatively about and to themselves. Examples of such statements include:

- "I'm stupid."
- "Everybody hates me."
- "I'm not good at anything."
- "Nobody cares if I'm alive."
- "I'm ugly."

Your child will also reveal his level of self-esteem through his behavior. Watch how he reacts to compliments, criticism, and defeat. Children with low self-esteem are uncomfortable with compliments. They do not believe the compliment is true and are therefore unwilling to accept it with a thank you. Instead they tend to break eye contact and shy away, either saying nothing or rejecting the compliment by berating themselves.

Children with low self-esteem have difficulty accepting negative feedback. Because their self-esteem is so fragile, the slightest indication that they have a fault stimulates a global sense of failure to which they react with anger.

Handling difficult tasks and failure also is very distressing for AD children with low self-esteem. Their frustration tolerance is very low and their temper flares rapidly if they are not immediately successful at a task.

Can a child have too much self-esteem?

Thinking too highly of yourself is not any better than thinking too little. When people think too highly of themselves we may label them as conceited, narcissistic, or egotistical. Just as adults can believe themselves to be more worthy than others view them, so too can children. AD children tend to be disliked by others, viewed as a know-it-all, condescending, and critical of others. Their adultlike manner of talking and advanced knowledge of certain subjects can give the impression of arrogance. The manner in which they do not respond to others can also give the impression that they believe they are superior to others.

AD children do have pockets of inflated self-worth, generally when they are displaying their expert knowledge on a topic of interest. Their impatience and intolerance for those who are less knowledgeable is indicative of their feelings of superiority. Unfortunately, they are alone in this feeling, as others find it offensive rather than impressive.

In all other areas of their functioning, however, AD children have little cause to feel more worthy than others. This may be the reason they cling to their special interest and are so intent on displaying their knowledge.

How will special education affect my child's self-esteem?

One of the first questions parents have when special education is recommended is "How will it affect my child's self-esteem?" Opinions are mixed as to whether or not special education has a positive, negative, or neutral effect on a child's self-esteem.

How your child's self-esteem is affected by special education will vary depending on the unique aspects of your child, her educational needs, and the individual aspects of the special education setting.

Assuming that special education has been recommended, you need to evaluate how your child is coping emotionally, socially, and behaviorally in the mainstream classroom. If she is frequently in trouble in the classroom, unable to follow rules, and rejected by her peers, chances are she has low self-esteem. If she remains in the same environment, she has little chance for changing the way she feels about herself. However, if she moves to a special education classroom that is structured for her to stay out of trouble, increases her ability to succeed in following the rules, and places her with similar peers with whom she can make friends, her self-esteem is likely to increase.

How can my child's teacher help with self-esteem?

A good portion of a negative sense of self has its roots on the school campus. Children with AD have difficulty getting through the school day without receiving negative feedback. Reprimands in the classroom and teasing on the playground contribute to low self-esteem.

Teachers can be of great help in your child's self-esteem with their praise and encouragement.

Ways your child's teacher can help include:

- Giving praise for effort
- Appointing your child as the classroom expert on a topic he excels in
- Creating a no-teasing rule in the classroom and on the playground
- Ensuring that teasers apologize to your child
- Assigning your child a special job to help him feel important
- Looking for ways to praise frequently
- Reading stories to the class that teach empathy and promote kindness
- Publicly praising your child to enhance him in the view of his classmates
- Creating a "You're a Star" program for students to write compliments on a paper star and hang on the classroom bulletin board
- Giving a weekly Friendship award to one student who exhibits true friendship
- Creating a compliment program for students to publicly praise one another in class

How does teasing affect self-esteem?

"Sticks and stones may break my bones, but words can never hurt me" is a familiar phrase every child learns early on to protect their self-esteem against the sting of teasing. Every child is teased at some point in their childhood. AD children are among the most teased and rejected students on campus. They suffer frequent name-calling and ridicule.

Unfortunately, AD children are also the most ill-equipped to cope with being teased. They lack the social skills to be able to respond appropriately. They may yell, cry, hit, and repeatedly tattle. Their immature responses cause more problems, often leading to more teasing, increased rejection, and consequences from parents and teachers.

For many adults with AD, the teasing they endured in school is flagged as a major cause of their suffering years later. Being called names, teased, bullied, and rejected hurts in the immediate moment and can hurt for days, months, and years later. It is thus critical that children with AD learn how to respond to teasing in the presence of their peers and learn how to cope with it internally so that it does not destroy their self-esteem.

How can I help my child cope with being teased?

One of children's biggest complaints about being teased is that adults do not do anything to help. Children are told to work it out themselves, yet they do not possess the knowledge, skills, or impulse control to do so.

They are also told to just ignore it. Any frequently teased child will tell you that ignoring simply does not work. Children who tease others can be relentless and have far more stamina in their teasing than your AD child has in ignoring.

Help your child understand that the reason he keeps getting teased is because he reacts. His reaction is like a jackpot on a slot machine, urging the teaser to keep going. Encourage your child not to be a reactor but instead to be a joiner. Joining in the teasing with laughter and agreement can stop the payoff the teaser is seeking.

Your child can disarm the teaser with some humorous phrases of agreement.

Some examples include:

- "Thank you for noticing!"
- "You got that right!"
- "You are so right!"
- "What can I say?"
- "I know—I wish I could be more like you!"
- "I can't argue with that!"
- "Don't I know it!"

Can extracurricular activities increase self-esteem?

School for many AD children represents an arena of failure and rejection that they cannot escape. Activities outside of school can provide an environment to preserve and enhance self-esteem.

Self-esteem found in other arenas can make up for the despondency many AD children feel at school. Success at an activity other than school can provide feelings of accomplishment, pride, and motivation. Outside activities can also provide an opportunity for your child to have positive interactions with other children.

Any outside activity that your child enjoys can increase self-esteem. It is the pleasure of the activity, not his ability, which generates self-esteem. Sports have been repeatedly shown to enhance self-esteem. Participants in athletic activities have better images of their own bodies, higher levels of self-esteem, and more trust for others. Girls in particular learn to appreciate their bodies and the fact that strength and endurance are assets. Participation in sports teaches children not just how to win, but how to lose. Sports teach children how to work with others and set goals.

Since children with AD often have poor motor skills and poor social skills, team sports are probably not the best arena for them. Individual sports of golf, gymnastics, track, and horseback riding provide benefits of sports without the stress of intense social interaction.

Can praise increase self-esteem?

Indiscriminate praise is meaningless. Praise is meaningful when it is based on your child's actual effort and performance. When children are praised regardless of how hard they tried or how much success they achieved, the praise becomes empty.

The purpose of praise is to engender positive feelings about oneself. The hope is that those positive feelings become part of your child's identity. When he is flattered about everything he has no way to form a realistic sense of self. He knows he is not good at everything and knows he does not put forth equal effort in everything he tries. If he is being positively reinforced for everything he does, he comes to disbelieve the praise, even when it is well-deserved.

Praise is important and feels good, but what really matters is how your child praises himself. He learns from your realistic feedback how to talk to himself about his good points and weak points, as well as his efforts. Your praise is most effective when it is truthful. Your child will mimic your praise when he is assessing himself in his mind. He will have a positive and accurate self-appraisal if you have helped him learn to evaluate his effort and performance in a realistic manner.

How can compliments increase my child's self-esteem?

Compliments make most people feel good about themselves. AD children are hungry for compliments but are often the least likely to receive them. The goal of compliments is to help your child feel competent and increase the chance he will repeat the behavior.

Compliments need to be truthful and genuine. False compliments can easily be detected by children—particularly those given by their parents. Compliment only when your child earns it with his effort or performance.

Since compliments belong to the receiver, they need to be about the receiver. Rather than telling your child how proud you are of him, tell him you hope he is proud of himself. You want him to be able to feel his own pride so that he will want to repeat the behavior and take pride in himself.

Make compliments only about praise, not an opportunity to teach, coach, or motivate. "You did a great job cleaning your room!" is only a compliment if you don't add, "Why can't you do it like this every time?"

How does my parenting style affect my child's self-esteem?

Authoritarian parents enforce rules but at the expense of their child's emotions. They use force and punishment to control their child, withdrawing and rejecting them when they disobey. These children tend to be anxious, withdrawn, and unhappy. Their social interactions are hostile and they are easily angered and defiant.

Permissive parents are nurturing but at the expense of imposing controls on their child. They allow their child to make decisions regardless of the child's ability to do so. These children have little structure and are permitted to behave as they choose. They tend to be behaviorally out-of-control, incapable of controlling their impulses, disobedient, and rebellious.

In contrast, parents who use an authoritative style have children that are happy, self-confident, and self-controlled. Authoritative parenting involves parents who make reasonable demands for behavior enforced by limit setting and insistence on obedience. Failure to obey consistently results in appropriate consequences. When their children are defiant, authoritative parents are patient and rational. They do not give in or respond harshly, but use reasonable, firm control with warmth and affection. Children raised by authoritative parents have increased chances for higher self-esteem, academic success, social maturity, and high moral achievement.

How can unconditional love help with self-esteem?

Almost every person desires acceptance by others. Those who are rejected become even needier. Imagine having no one in your life who accepts you the way you are. Each encounter you have in your life leaves you with the feeling that you are different, cause problems, and frustrate others, causing them to not want to be around you.

It is immeasurably helpful for your child to have a safe haven to come home to. Knowing when he gets home he will be accepted and loved can help him get through a tough day at school. A home where he knows he is accepted for who he is, with all his symptoms and quirks, provides a safe harbor from the harshness of life outside the home.

If your child has significant symptoms, you can be sure he is not getting unconditional acceptance outside the home, so you must be sure to give it in the home. If you do not give him unconditional love, then who will?

If you accept him and he feels this, he will come to accept and love himself and search for this in others. He learns that despite his symptoms, he is worthy.

Can helping others increase my child's self-esteem?

It is human nature to want to help others. Helping another person can engender great feelings of competence, pride, self-worth, and satisfaction, feelings your child likely does not find at school.

There are many places where your child can volunteer to help others. Many schools have created programs for AD students to help. Since many AD children get along much better with younger children, they can find opportunities to be a teacher's helper in kindergarten and first-grade classrooms. Reading to the class, tutoring, or playing games with the younger students can give the AD child a sense of competence. He will also be in an environment where he is liked, he is admired, and the children are excited to see him.

Even though AD children might be rejected by their peers, they are often adored by adults. Your child can receive positive feedback from visiting retirement and nursing homes. He can read to the residents, bring a therapy dog, entertain them with a talent, or play board games. He will learn about kindness toward others while receiving positive feedback from grateful seniors who may otherwise be without the joy that a child brings.

How can I help my child stop negative self-talk?

We all have an internal voice we use to talk to ourselves. This self-talk is how we give ourselves feedback. We each have statements we are prone to repeat to ourselves over and over, as if we make a tape recording and press play repeatedly. Children with high self-esteem have positive self-talk. Those with low self-esteem and/or depression engage in more negative self-talk.

You are likely to hear your child criticize himself. When you hear your child say something such as "I'm stupid," instead of telling him he is wrong, a more helpful approach is to help him talk about why he feels this way. Once he explains the situation that is causing him to feel stupid, you will be able to offer a more reality-based counterstatement. You may respond with, "Sounds more like you feel you are bad at book reports, not that you are stupid." This helps put his negative self-talk in a more realistic perspective. He may indeed be poor at writing book reports, something he will have to work on, but he is not altogether stupid. Eventually he will learn to have this type of realistic talk within himself.

How can I help my child accept his weaknesses?

Parents sometimes make the mistake of trying to make their child feel he is good at everything. This false feedback will result in your child having a distorted sense of self. Children need to learn to appraise themselves accurately.

When your child expresses negative self-talk that is accurate, it can be helpful to assist him in accepting the negative aspect of himself. If your child is truly poor at kickball, there are several responses that may be of help. "Would you like to be better at kickball?" shows him that the situation might be temporary. "Is it important to you to be good at kickball?" prompts him to realize he does not have to be good at everything. "Is there something you feel that you are really good at?" helps him change the focus from the negative to the positive. Offering these concepts in question form is better than simply telling him that he does not have to be good at everything, or that he shouldn't worry because he is good at swimming. Questions teach him the process of evaluating himself and his negative self-talk so that eventually he can do it on his own.

How do I give my child a realistic sense of self?

As a parent, you have a dramatic effect on your child's self-esteem. Your encouragement when she is discouraged provides a temporary voice that tells her to keep going until she is able to tell that to herself. Every child must master the emotions of defeat, being able to persevere when things get tough, and keeping coming back despite failure. Children with a realistic sense of self do not become shattered when they do not succeed and are able to use self-talk to soothe their upset feelings.

Your child will develop a realistic sense of self from mirroring what you tell her. Honest feedback is what works. Praise in times of success is easy. It is in times of defeat that it is most difficult to help your child maintain her self-esteem. Some reality-based encouraging words might include, "I know you are disappointed, but…

- you sure looked like you were really trying hard."
- you put forth a really good effort and that's what really counts."
- it's the fun of it that is important, not the outcome."
- you can be proud of yourself for hanging in there."
- you are handling your upset really well."

How do I help my child find a sense of competence?

We all need to feel that we are competent at something. The more things your child feels good about doing the more feelings of competence she will have, leading to increased self-esteem.

Your child will likely have a sense of competence related to her special interest. Her feelings of competence are probably well-deserved, as there are probably few others with her knowledge. The challenge for the AD child is to encourage her to share her competence with others in a way that is inviting. Finding a club for her special interest provides fun, competence, and a chance to share it with others.

Find opportunities to point out to your child the things she is good at. She does not have to earn the first-place ribbon in an art contest to feel competent. She can feel competent that she consistently shows up for her lessons, paints something new each class, and is good at mixing colors. Look for all the ways she is good, not just the obvious. Your verbal recognition will eventually be replaced by her own self-acknowledgment.

Your child can also be competent in character traits. She need not have a talent or skill to experience competence. She can feel good about being honest, trustworthy, a loyal friend, or someone who helps others in need.

How can Snapshots enhance my child's self-esteem?

Snapshots are moments where your child shines above his usual functioning. They are moments of increased feelings of competence. Starting with show-and-tell in kindergarten, teachers use Snapshots to create opportunities for each child to stand out in a positive light. School plays, track meets, awards ceremonies, and certificates of accomplishment are familiar Snapshots schools create to showcase their students and provide opportunities for feelings of enhanced esteem.

AD children need numerous Snapshots to sustain their feelings of self-worth in between the big events. Work with your child's teacher to find ways for your child to experience additional Snapshots. Create opportunities for your child to display a particular talent or interest in his class and perhaps other classrooms. Mentioning your child's unique talent, interest, or experience in the school newspaper gives public recognition, good feelings for him, and a trinket for his scrapbook of accomplishments.

What can I do to improve my child's self-esteem?

People with high self-esteem have a variety of abilities that allow them to remain feeling positive about themselves regardless of the challenges they face, the failures they experience, or the criticism they receive. Abilities you can foster in your child to work toward increasing self-esteem include:

- Willingness to try new experiences
- Using positive self-talk
- Confidence to try
- Ability to accept compliments
- Comfort with the reality that he cannot be good at everything
- Perseverance when things get tough
- Belief in himself that if he keeps trying, he has a chance for success
- Feeling comfortable saying, "I'm not good at…"
- Focusing on what he is good at instead of what he is not
- Separating areas of weakness from overall worthiness
- Understanding that criticism does not mean he is a failure
- Not fearing failure
- Measuring success based on effort, fun, and experience rather than the outcome
- Having multiple self-esteems

Chapter 12

GROWING UP WITH ASPERGER'S

- What impact does Asperger's Disorder have during adolescence?
- What impact does Asperger's Disorder have during college years?
- What impact does Asperger's Disorder have during adult years?
- What impact does Asperger's Disorder have on employment?
- What problems does Asperger's Disorder cause on the job?
- Should employers be told about Asperger's Disorder?
- Can Asperger's Disorder be an asset on the job?
- How does Asperger's Disorder impact dating relationships?
- How does Asperger's Disorder impact adolescent sexuality?
- How does Asperger's Disorder impact adult sexuality?
- How does Asperger's Disorder impact marriage?
- Are adults with Asperger's Disorder prone to psychological problems?
- Are teens and adults with Asperger's Disorder prone to use drugs and alcohol?
- Are teens and adults with Asperger's Disorder prone to crime?
- What should I know about the criminal justice system and Asperger's Disorder?
- What can parents do to ensure a good future for their child?
- Can Asperger's Disorder be a strength?
- What is the good news about Asperger's Disorder?
- Can Asperger's Disorder be a gift?

What impact does Asperger's Disorder have during adolescence?

The biggest impact AD has during the teen years is on social relationships. During adolescence, fitting in and making friends is of utmost importance. The social abnormalities of childhood become more apparent in adolescence. As friendships mature into sharing, caring, and trusting, the AD teen's inability to participate in deeper relationships becomes more obvious to her peers. It is during this phase in life that teens with AD begin to gain deeper awareness that they are not accepted and do not fit in with a peer group. Sadness, low self-esteem, and even depression can be the result. While this sounds bleak, it can actually be the hopeful beginning of your teen taking a closer look at her social interactions and working harder to use more effective social skills.

The good news about AD during adolescence is that AD teens are less likely to act out. Compared to their peers, especially those with other disorders, AD teens have less rebellion and antisocial behaviors. Being outside a peer group and being oblivious to peer pressure and the latest trend may actually turn out to be a good thing that provides a protective barrier to doing what everyone else at school is doing.

What impact does Asperger's Disorder have during college years?

The majority of teens with AD graduate from high school and many go on to college. There is nothing about having AD that specifically prevents one from graduating college. However, many challenges can be faced with the independence of living away from home. Getting up on time for class, managing the workload, being offered drugs and alcohol, managing money, dating, and sex can be more challenging for the AD student than her nondisordered peers. These aspects of college are usually more stressful than learning the academic material. The high level of structure and assistance the student had at home and school during childhood and adolescence is suddenly non-existent when she gets to college.

While federal law dictates that all colleges must comply with Section 504 of the Rehabilitation Act, these modifications and accommodations can only address so much. Most colleges are not prepared to meet the vast social and emotional needs that AD students have. However, as more and more students with AD attend college, special programs to help them succeed are being developed on college campuses. Studies are finding that college students who have contact with a counselor or mentor on a daily basis are finding less stress, better coping abilities, and greater success remaining in college.

What impact does Asperger's Disorder have during adult years?

AD is a lifetime disorder. Symptoms will remain throughout adult years. How severely the adult is impacted depends largely on how severe the symptoms were during childhood and adolescence. Outcome is also somewhat dependent on IQ, with those having the highest IQ having a better outcome. The level of services received during childhood and adolescence is also expected to have a role in outcome, with more intensive and longer-term services predicting a better outcome. A good overall outcome is generally defined as having some meaningful friendships, being employed or in job training, being responsible for one's own finances, and living independently.

AD will impact each adult in a different way. Each adult, in turn, will be impacted more severely in some areas than others. Outcome research for AD is a recent area of study lacking strong statistics at the present time. Adults with AD may not have been diagnosed in childhood, may have been diagnosed with autism as a child, and/or may not have received any services during their childhood and teens years. These factors combine to make knowledge of the real outcome of AD difficult to know.

What impact does Asperger's Disorder have on employment?

The limited information that is available about the future employment for individuals with AD is a mixture of good and bad news. The good news is that AD adults are fully employable. Their skills in job tasks are usually very good and if they find a career in their area of interest they can be very successful. The bad news is that their social difficulties interfere with their ability to keep jobs. In fact, social difficulties on the job are the leading cause of job failure for adults with AD.

While the job market is wide open to individuals with AD, there are certain careers where they are more likely to find long-term success. The ideal career has very limited social contact with people and a high level of independent work. Jobs that focus on task completion rather than customer service would suit many adults with AD. Careers in computers, accounting, engineering, drafting, mechanics, laboratory, and the Internet are ideal, as they maximize skills but minimize social interaction.

Oftentimes a special interest develops into a career and what may have seemed odd to others during his childhood has the potential to give the adult with AD something many adults never have—a true passion for their career.

What problems does Asperger's Disorder cause on the job?

Interviews are often the first job difficulty faced by those with AD. Their unusual language and poor ability to interact with others may result in failure to get hired despite having the necessary skills. An employment counselor or therapist can provide training and rehearsal in interviewing skills.

Once on the job, those with AD report having trouble keeping their positions. They describe that the social skills required to function in the work setting are just too overwhelming. They report it is easier to work in smaller settings with fewer people to deal with and less activity and confusion going on. Even with small work environments, the AD adult finds that too much of his mental and emotional energy is spent trying to interpret the words and behaviors of his coworkers, as well as trying to make sure he makes the correct choice about his own words and actions. Some report not knowing what topics are acceptable to talk about and what topics are considered inappropriate. It is like working in a foreign country where you only speak a little bit of the language and know only a few of the customs. The amount of effort it takes to navigate the social arena of a job interferes with actually doing the job.

Job Difficulties
- Finding work at level of education/ability
- Keeping a job long-term
- Getting along with coworkers
- Sensory overload
- Coping with the unpredictable
- Learning unwritten rules of the job
- Failing to ask for help or clarification
- Socially inappropriate behavior
- Misinterpreting others' words/actions
- Easily frustrated
- Multitasking
- Time management
- Presenting well in interview

- Inability to work in a group
- Inflexibility
- Need for excessively precise expectations
- Poor organization
- Difficulty remembering verbal instructions

Should employers be told about Asperger's Disorder?

There are pros and cons to disclosing to an employer that you have AD. Some AD teens and adults believe if they tell the employer during the interview, they will not get the job. Those who have followed this practice, however, warn that once they are hired they are faced with having to hide their symptoms from their coworkers and it is usually not long before their difficulties are apparent to their coworkers and supervisor. Those who have disclosed their AD to the interviewer report being happy they had done so, as once they started the job their employer was able to give them what they needed to do the job successfully.

The potential assets and liabilities of disclosure should be carefully considered for each job interview. Discussing and rehearsing disclosure with an employment counselor or therapist is a good idea. Be clear about the reasons for disclosure and what is needed from the employer if a job offer is made. If disclosure is decided against, the job candidate can prepare questions ahead of time to determine if the job will meet his needs for success. Again, an employment counselor or therapist can help with the phrasing of these questions.

Adults with AD report greater success in their job with the following:

- **Job mentor or coach:** An established coworker who can answer questions instead of trying to figure it out alone.
- **Clear expectations:** Written details of rules, routine, duties,

procedures, and requirements for productivity that tell what, when, where, and how to do the job.

- **Organization:** Additional time to organize before starting tasks.
- **Increased time to learn the job:** Additional time to learn the job before being considered for termination.
- **Similar coworkers:** Working with others who are similar decreases social difficulties.
- **Interest-focused jobs:** Finding work in an area of interest.
- **Preparation:** Being notified of upcoming changes in tasks, procedures, schedules, etc.
- **Written information:** Information in writing increases success more than verbal information.
- **Limited social contact:** Less contact with people will decrease social difficulties.
- **Supervisors:** Clear expectations and being left alone to do the work without micromanagement. Accepting and tolerant supervisor.
- **Environment:** Quiet and away from coworkers.
- **Teamwork:** None or very limited.

Can Asperger's Disorder be an asset on the job?

Having AD can be a great asset if the adult finds his way into the right position. Several aspects of AD that cause problems in the social arena can be ideal traits as an employee. The lack of interpersonal connectedness makes the AD worker more connected to his job than the average employee. Many adults with AD label themselves as workaholics. They love their work and derive much of their life's satisfaction from their jobs. Their lack of interest in social relationships and people's emotions and opinions leaves the AD adult out of the troublesome office politics, gossip, and conflicts that detract his coworkers from getting the job done. If given specific procedures, duties, deadlines, and a quiet environment to do his job alone, the AD adult will be a valuable employee. Dedication to the job, perfectionism, and attention to detail render high performance and little time lost due to errors. His preference for routine in his life will yield a reliable employee who shows up to work daily and can be counted on to do his duties day in and day out. Provided he feels comfortable in his work environment, the AD adult can be a long-term employee.

Job strengths found in employees with AD
- Punctual
- Attention to detail
- Comfort with repetitive tasks
- Rarely bored
- Loyal to the job
- Longevity if not fired
- Follow procedures consistently
- Do not break known company rules
- Rare absences
- Rare personal phone calls
- Avoid office politics, cliques, and gossip
- Will not waste time socializing
- Creative
- Think outside the box
- Single-minded focus on work
- Excellent memory
- Love to work
- Content to work alone

How does Asperger's Disorder impact dating relationships?

The dating life of teens with AD is rather limited if not nonexistent. While they have the same wants and desires as any teen, their social deficits prevent them from dating. Teens and adults report that they cannot tell if someone is rejecting them politely or flirting to show interest. An adolescent boy with AD may pursue a girl until her parents have to put a stop to it because he does not understand her polite attempts to tell him she is not interested. Others miss out on opportunities to ask for a date because they cannot recognize signs of interest.

The social skills of the adult world and the dating world are much more subtle than the skills they used during childhood and adolescence, and many adults with AD describe that instead of getting easier in adulthood, dating actually becomes more difficult. Other than knowing not to ask out a married person or someone in a relationship, they do not know how to judge who is an appropriate choice for a date. While many AD adults do date, a large percentage has never dated.

Once dating begins, the difficulty AD teens and adults have with expressing emotions and sharing feelings is a barrier to advancing beyond dating. Loneliness and depression often emerge in the young adult years as the result of the inability to date and establish a close relationship.

How does Asperger's Disorder impact adolescent sexuality?

While their development of sexuality is equal to their peers, teens with AD are found to have less sexual knowledge than their non-disordered counterparts. They are sexually immature, with some researchers reporting a five-year delay in sexual maturity. They engage in more inappropriate sexual behavior, including touching others, touching their own private body parts in public, and publicly talking about sex in ways that are inappropriate compared to the ways their peers talk about sex. They are less aware of rules for privacy, such as knocking on closed doors and not removing their clothing in public. Social skills deficits are believed to be the primary cause of these sexual problems.

Parents of AD teens report greater worry about their adolescent's sexual behavior than do parents of nondisordered teens. The older the teen becomes the greater the parents' worries. Despite parents reporting that they provided their child with sexual education, they nonetheless report concerns that their teen does not know proper sexual behavior.

These findings emphasize the need to provide AD children with a solid foundation of social skills training in childhood followed by specific instructions on dating and making romantic physical contact, as well as sex education.

How does Asperger's Disorder impact adult sexuality?

Behaviors of engaging in inappropriate sexual behavior and disregarding privacy during adolescent years disappear by adulthood. What remains, however, is awkwardness in interacting in dating situations. Despite having sexual education, adults with AD report they do not know how to incorporate that information in the dating world. Their desires for physical intimacy are reported to be equal to nondisordered adults; however, they are often unsuccessful in establishing romantic relationships that lead to sexual contact. Young adults with AD are found to express dissatisfaction with their sexual life. Surveys of single adults with AD find that only a small percentage report having any sexual experience. They do not know how to read the subtle social cues of their dates and are unable to tell whether or not physical affection will be welcomed. The unspoken language of dating and sexuality is incredibly difficult for them to read. Many simply give up after a few negative experiences that reinforce their belief that they have no clue how to tell who is interested and who is just being polite. Those adults who do establish sexual relationships are no different than their nondisordered counterparts, indicating that it is not the physical aspects of sexuality that are troublesome, but the social.

How does Asperger's Disorder impact marriage?

Unfortunately, there are no statistics to tell us how many adults with AD marry.

For every article that reports AD adults marry at the same rate as non-AD adults, there is a research survey that reports less than 5 percent ever marry. The vast number of social problems would suggest that marriage may not be in the future for some.

For those that do marry, there are unique challenges for the non-AD spouse. The enduring symptoms of AD can make a close relationship difficult, particularly if the spouse does not understand the disorder. Spouses are likely to use the terms self-centered, obsessive, and rigid to describe their AD partner. Emotional closeness is often lacking in these marriages as well. The non-AD spouse may feel as if she is not cared about and that the relationship is one-sided, with her putting forth all the effort for communicating, expressing feelings, and discussing problems. The non-AD spouse may feel left out of the AD spouse's special interest. Attempts to have a shared experience are met with a dull, unenthusiastic response. The non-AD spouse is usually the social chairman and the representative of the family, leaving the AD spouse free from the stress of interpersonal communication.

Are adults with Asperger's Disorder prone to psychological problems?

Depression is by far the most common psychological disorder experienced by adults with AD, probably accounting for about 40 percent of secondary disorders. Depression can begin at any point in life. Children can be depressed, but more often it appears during adolescence and adulthood. Adults with AD experience frequent depression, most often due to loneliness.

Anxiety is the second most common disorder experienced by adults with AD. Their difficulty in social interactions can make them so nervous that they develop social phobia. A more general form of anxiety, called generalized anxiety disorder, is experienced as frequent and uncontrollable worrying about various aspects of daily life.

Still other adults with AD may not have severe enough anxiety to have a full disorder, but nonetheless experience bouts of anxiousness. During these episodes it is not uncommon to see a rise in the need for routine. Major life changes can also result in high levels of anxiety, agitation, unpredictable behavior, increased rituals, and confusion.

Adults with AD may have some obsessive thoughts and compulsive behaviors as part of the disorder. However, some adults have repetitive thoughts and rituals that are uncontrollable, distressing, and severe enough to be a secondary diagnosis of Obsessive-Compulsive Disorder (OCD).

Are teens and adults with Asperger's Disorder prone to use drugs and alcohol?

In general, teens and adults with psychological disorders are at higher risk for abusing drugs and alcohol than their nondisordered peers. Fortunately this does not seem to be the case for AD. Drugs and alcohol seem to hold little interest for the majority of teens and adults with AD. It is not clear why this is the case, but mental health professionals guess that the social isolation that AD teens experience may prevent them from being exposed to drugs and alcohol by their peers. Additional prevention factors might also include the lack of need for excitement and sensation-seeking that is characteristic of AD.

When alcohol and drugs are used, it is most often a form of self-medicating a secondary disorder. Depression can feel less intense while intoxicated. Social phobia can be temporarily decreased when drugs give a sense of confidence. The short-term relief that substances provide from the symptoms of depression and/or anxiety can quickly create a reinforcing cycle where the teen and adult with AD learns that he feels better when under the influence. The obsessional tendency of AD increases the chance that once substances are used with any regularity, they may easily become abused.

Are teens and adults with Asperger's Disorder prone to crime?

There seems to be little relationship between AD and criminal activity. When crimes are committed by individuals with AD, they have a different flavor than crimes committed by other disordered offenders. While their criminal activity may result in harm to people or property, it is usually not their intent to do so. Instead, their criminal behavior is often motivated by their special interest. For example, a teen interested in chemistry may experiment with explosives and bring them to school to see how they explode in a locker. In other cases, the criminal behavior may be related to a coexisting disorder rather than AD, such as a depressed teen who assaults a schoolmate who relentlessly teases him.

Other criminal behavior may be the result of misunderstanding appropriate rules of behavior, such as following a romantic interest home repeatedly. What seems to the AD adult to be a display of interest appears to be stalking to the victim. Teens with AD may naively engage in criminal activity at the urging of their peers. In stark contrast to most criminal offenders, those with AD do not try to cover up their crimes and will readily admit to their behaviors when questioned.

What should I know about the criminal justice system and Asperger's Disorder?

Knowing that some teens and adults with AD may be vulnerable to criminal behavior as a result of their disorder, parents need to take a higher level of involvement in their teen and adult child's life. Repeated education about the rules of appropriate behavior is necessary, as is a close level of supervision.

All children, teens, and adults with AD should have an ID card or bracelet that identifies them as having AD, along with contact information. Police will likely notice that your child is different. However, they probably will not recognize that he has a serious disorder and therefore will not treat him any differently. Individuals with AD are not likely to grasp the situation they are in when being questioned by police. They may not be able to understand the consequences of their words and behavior. Their distorted perceptions of themselves and others may result in their making statements that are inaccurate but nonetheless incriminating. Their difficulty in social relationships may prevent them from understanding the formal relationships between themselves and police. Should your child be charged with a crime, it is important to seek advice from professionals experienced with AD.

What can parents do to ensure a good future for their child?

Every parent wants his child to be happy and have a successful life. As a parent of an AD child, you have a far greater challenge than other parents. You are the key to your child's happiness and success.

The more help you provide your child, the greater his chance for a happy childhood and adolescence and a good future as an adult. You have a responsibility to do all you can for your child. Having a child with AD means sacrificing time, effort, emotions, and money to give him the best life possible.

As a parent of an AD child, the first step to take to help your child is to acknowledge the difficulty you are faced with and accept that you need professional guidance. You are not expected to know how to raise a child with a disorder. There is no shame in getting help— only in refusing to admit that you need it.

What AD Children Need	What AD Children Might Need
Thorough evaluation for AD	Special education
Thorough evaluation for other disorders	Individual psychotherapy
Behavior modification	Occupational therapy
Social skills training	Family therapy
Anger management training	Medication
Emotional regulation training	IQ testing
Extracurricular activities	Academic achievement testing

Can Asperger's Disorder be a strength?

Despite the large number of problems that necessitate therapy and training, AD does not have to be completely negative. Some children and teens with AD are able to embrace their symptoms and find the unique benefits the disorder offers. When parents and children can change their perspective, some of the symptoms of AD can become assets to be harnessed instead of symptoms to try to eliminate.

AD children have a very unique way of perceiving things. They think of things no one else could possibly entertain. Today's business model of "thinking outside the box" is made for the AD person.

While schools may not value the entrepreneurial spirit of AD, there are many arenas outside of school that do.

List the symptoms your child displays and consider how each might be channeled into a talent, hobby, or strength. The tendency to talk incessantly about a special interest and show off knowledge can be helpful in tutoring younger students in the favorite subject. Socially isolated children who find solace in books can make social connections in a book club.

Turning a symptom into strength can change the way you respond to your child. Your child will find increased happiness and esteem from this approach.

What is the good news about Asperger's Disorder?

The future of your child might seem somewhat bleak when you first glance at some of the research findings. Underemployment, social isolation, failure to live independently, and depression can paint a grim outlook. Meant to inform rather than depress you as a parent, these findings provide you with the reality of what can happen to your child. These findings should prompt you into action to obtain all the services your child needs and to stick with them for as long as he displays symptoms.

While some of the research findings bring bad news, many studies bring good news. Most teens and adults with AD:

- Graduate high school
- Are not rebellious
- Do not fall for peer pressure
- Abstain from using drugs
- Abstain from abusing alcohol
- Respect rules and laws
- Do not engage in criminal behavior
- Have a good work ethic

Can Asperger's Disorder be a gift?

It's all in how you look at it. The more you and your child can view the symptoms in a positive way the less negative impact the disorder will have. Your child's qualities and his day-to-day life actually sound rather pleasant if you view you child's symptoms as a gift.

Trait	Gift
Obsessive	Passionate
Intensive	Objective
Rule-bound	Moral and ethical
Unemotional	Stoic
Rigid	Predictable
Inflexible	Precise
Loner	Comfortable being alone
Eccentric	Interesting
Limited interests	Focused and committed to his interests
Shows off knowledge	Informative
Cannot read social cues	Others can be open and direct with him
Ritualistic	Will not be bored with repetitive tasks
Odd thoughts	Creative
Limited self-awareness	Free from self-consciousness
Lack of insight	Free from preoccupation with own faults
Excessively detailed	Finds entertainment in the mundane things
Repeats the same mistakes	Not plagued with guilt for mistakes
Selfish	Gets own needs met
Talks too much	Excited to share ideas and interests

THE 5 MOST IMPORTANT LISTS YOU NEED

What are the ten questions you must ask your doctor about diagnosis?

1. Is AD an area of specialty for you?
2. What procedures do you use to evaluate for AD?
3. Do you think all children need to have formal testing to be evaluated?
4. Will you use psychological testing? If so, what tests and what is the purpose?
5. Do you use medical tests? If so, what tests and what is the purpose?
6. What sources of information do you use to make your diagnosis?
7. How do you determine ordinary behavior from AD?
8. What other disorders have will you consider besides AD?
9. Will your review my child's school records?
10. Are there indications that my child should be tested for learning disorders?

What are ten coexisting disorders your doctor must consider?

1. Attention Deficit Disorder (ADD)
2. Attention Deficit Hyperactivity Disorder (ADHD)
3. Learning Disorders
4. Depression
5. Anxiety
6. Oppositional Defiant Disorder
7. Obsessive-Compulsive Disorder
8. Bipolar Disorder
9. Tourette's Syndrome
10. Social Phobia

What are ten things you must tell your child's doctor?

1. Problems with eye contact
2. Preferences for being alone
3. Ability to play and get along with other children
4. Ability to use imagination when playing alone or with others
5. Time spent playing, talking, and learning about special interests
6. Ability to converse with others
7. Insistence on routine and sameness
8. Insistence on repeating certain behaviors or rituals
9. Sensitivities to sensations of sound, taste, smell, touch, or visual stimulation
10. Ability to walk, run, throw, catch, jump, use pencil, button clothing, etc.

What are ten things you must tell your child's teacher?

1. That your child has AD
2. Whether or not your child has other diagnoses
3. Whether or not your child has any learning disorders
4. If your child is from a divorced family
5. If your child has sensory sensitivities
6. What behavior problems can be expected in the classroom
7. What behavior problems can be expected on the playground
8. What rewards your child is motivated to work for
9. What consequences are effective in decreasing inappropriate behavior
10. What special talents, hobbies, and interests your child has

What are ten parenting techniques you must use?
1. Structured routine
2. Rule notebook
3. Predictable consequences
4. Consistency
5. Positive reinforcement
6. Shaping
7. Behavior chart
8. Time-out
9. Contracts
10. Functional Behavioral Analysis

SECTION 504 ACCOMMODATIONS AND MODIFICATIONS

Section 504 Accommodations and Modifications

This chart may be used in several ways. You may use it to prepare for your Section 504 meeting by identifying which symptoms your child has that interfere with his ability to benefit from his education. Review the list of possible accommodations and modifications and choose those that you feel may be of help to your child. Bring this checklist with you to your meeting as a worksheet when working with your child's education team.

If you are not seeking 504 Accommodations and Modifications but would like to work with your child's teacher to implement a few of the ideas that follow you may bring this worksheet with you to your parent-teacher conference as a tool you both can use to find solutions.

Whether or not your child has Section 504, use this worksheet for yourself, following the same steps of identifying the symptoms and implementing some of the suggested accommodations and modifications at home. These techniques work anywhere, not just in the classroom.

Finally, you may use this chart in your work with your child's psychologist. Learning how to execute many of these techniques is easier said than done. Professional guidance can help you fine tune your skills and allow you to successfully and rapidly find success.

Try to select a realistic number of techniques. Try as you might, it would be impossible to do them all! Focus on one to three techniques until you have them solidly in place before adding more. Over time you will be able to employ many of these techniques to structure how you work with your child and her school work. As she matures, changes from grade to grade, and circumstances change, you will need to modify the techniques you use to fit her level of functioning and her unique home and school situation.

Language Characteristics	Interventions
Irrelevant comments	Prompt to say something about topic
Interrupts	Red-yellow-green light to cue to wait or talk
Talks only about special interest	Limit the time child can talk about interest
Difficulty understanding complex language	Interpret/use simple language
Difficulty following directions	Check understanding/provide written directions
Difficulty understanding double entendres	Provide explanation
Interprets literally what is said	Provide explanation
Slow to respond to questions	Give time to answer
Difficulty understanding sarcasm/humor	Provide explanation
	Watch comedies
	Read children's joke books
Starts over again when interrupted	Try to avoid interrupting
Difficulty understanding abstract concepts	Use concrete language
	Provide explanation
Talks "at" you, not "with" you	Prompt to let others take turn
Talks loudly	Prompt to use inside or quiet voice
Unusual voice tone—robotic, mechanical	Speech therapy
Dominates class discussion	Announce how many questions will be allowed
	Prompt student to let others have a turn

Dominates class discussion continued	Prompt student to "hold that thought"
	Praise for being patient
	Prompt to wait for turn
	Provide empathy about waiting being difficult

Sensory Sensitivities	Helpful Tips
Auditory sensitivity	Make a list of sounds that cause distress
	Eliminate sounds if possible
	Listen to music to cover sounds
	Earplugs to decrease sound
	Relaxation techniques to decrease upset
	Allow retreat to a quiet place
	Keep level of sound low
	Occupational therapy to decrease sensitivity
	Warn of upcoming noises
Tactile sensitivity	Make a list of materials that cause distress
	Make a list of types of touch that cause distress
	Eliminate materials that cause distress
	Avoid touch that causes distress
	Occupational therapy to decrease sensitivity
	Ask permission to touch child
	Warn child if you are going to touch

Visual sensitivity	Make a list of visual items that cause distress
	Eliminate visual items that cause distress
	Avoid visual items that cause distress
	Allow use of sunglasses when needed
	Use low lights when possible
Gustatory/Olfactory sensitivity	Make a list of smells that cause distress
	Make a list of foods that cause distress
	Eliminate foods and smells that cause distress
	Avoid foods and smells that cause distress
	Warn when foods and smells will be present
	Allow child to reject foods that cause distress
	Occupational therapy if serious problems

Need for Routine and Sameness	Helpful Tips
Insistence on routines	Provide consistent daily routine
	Post daily schedule on wall
	Use pictures on daily schedule
	Understanding and tolerant teacher
Negative reactions to change in environment	Keep physical environment the same
	Avoid surprises
	Provide an organized environment

Resists change	Prepare ahead for upcoming change
	Story boards to cope with upcoming change
	Use pictures to show upcoming change
	Slowly expose to new settings/activities
Difficulty with unstructured time	Schedule activities to fill in unstructured time
Difficulty with transitions	Supervise during transitions (e.g., recess, lunch)
	Give warnings 10, 5, and 1 minute prior
	Minimize transitions
	Remind rules for behavior during transitions
	Assign buddy during transitions
	Help select activity during transition
	Define consequences for misbehavior
	Praise appropriate behavior
	Create reward system for appropriate behavior

Emotional Characteristics	Helpful Tips
Difficulty reading the emotions of others	Use pictures to teach facial expressions
	Movie therapy
	Social skills therapy
Inflexibility	Rehearse in advance upcoming changes
	Offer choices
	Avoid power struggle

Low self-esteem	Look for opportunities to praise
	Point out what he does well
	Compliment her strengths
	Provide opportunities to feel competent
	Watch for depression that requires therapy
Difficulty tolerating making mistakes	Teach positive self-talk
	Teach self-soothing techniques
	Encourage self-acceptance
	Encourage child to move on to next task
	Remind that mistakes are acceptable
Temper outbursts	Provide safe place to retreat
	Catch it early and diffuse
	Stop all demands on child until calm
	Withdraw if caught in power struggle
	Teach self-soothing techniques
Easily overwhelmed	Provide consistent daily schedule
	Teach positive self-talk ("I can do this")
	Eliminate obvious stressors
	Look for signs of stress and reduce quickly
	Assign adult support person to see one time daily
	Teach deep breathing
	Teach muscle relaxation
	Teach counting backwards
	Teach visualizing happy images
	Provide safe place to retreat

Motor-Skills Characteristics	Helpful Tips
Poor coordination	Involve in fitness activities
	Provide play time
	Occupational therapy
	Protect student from teasing on playground
	Do not grade on sports ability
	Provide alternative athletic activities
Prefers individual to team sports	Do not push team sports
	Provide activities until favorite is found
	Do fitness activities (e.g., gym, swim, bike)
Poor handwriting	Allow extra time on writing tasks
	Allow computer in place of writing
	Occupational therapy
	Use paper with writing guidelines
	Enroll in art class
	Use stencils to practice letters
	Use stencils for art to improve pen/pencil use
	Use tracing paper to improve pen/pencil use
	Allow use of wide-lined paper
	Grade for content, not writing technique
	Allow printing instead of handwriting

Academic Characteristics	Helpful Tips
Average to above-average intelligence	Mainstream classroom
Trouble with directions given aloud	Give simple directions
	Breaking directions down into simple steps
	Speak slowly
	Repeat directions
	Check for understanding of directions
	Do not assume child understood just because he parrots back what he has heard
	Provide written directions on index cards
	Provide written directions on chalkboard
	Ask child to explain directions in his own words
Poor problem solving	Provide direct instruction on problem solving
Comprehension problems	Explain concepts
	Avoid verbal overload
Excellent memory for facts	Provide opportunity to demonstrate memory
Poor motivation if not interested	Create activity-based learning where possible
	Set firm expectation even if not interested
	Break down tasks into smaller steps or present it another way
	Show examples of what is required
	Offer added explanation and try to simplify when lesson concepts are abstract
	Offer reward of free time for work completed

Good at mathematical computations	Match math assignments with math skills
Begins to read early	Match reading assignments with reading skills
Difficulty listening and taking notes	Provide a copy of lecture notes
	Emphasize and review main points
	Allow sharing of notes with another student
Difficulty listening and copying board	Provide a copy of lecture notes
	Allow sharing of notes with another student
	Emphasize and review main points
Visual learner	Use picture cues
Poor organization	Teach organization tools
	Teach how to use an outline
	Helps prioritize assignments
	Provide written list of what to do in what order
	Praise for proper organization
	Establish weekly notebook checks
Disrupts class	Seat near teacher
	Catch child being good and praise
	Use hand signal to prompt child to remain quiet
	Use behavior chart for proper behavior
	Ignore minor misbehavior
	Teach how to get attention appropriately
	Redirect child toward appropriate behavior

Social Skills Characteristics	Helpful Tips
Poor eye contact	Don't assume no eye contact = not listening
	Don't force eye contact
	Those with AD think better without eye contact
	Say, "Thank you for looking at me"
	Prompt, "Can you look at me?" but don't insist
Easy target for bullying	Assign a play buddy on playground
	No bullying policy on campus
	Educate class about disabilities
	Model acceptance, kindness, and patience
	Teach acceptance, kindness, and patience
	Praise students who stick up for peers
	Create weekly friendship award
	Showcase AD child's abilities
	Supervise playground and hallways
	Teach peers how to respond to AD child's behavior
	Protect child from bullying
Cannot read social cues	Seat child next to kind student
	Use story boards
	Use comic strip conversations
	Social skills group therapy
	Movie therapy
	Explain social cues
	Point out social cues to child and explain
	Prompt to guess what social cue means

Does not understand rules of social interaction	Prompt to guess what social cue means
	Teach rules repeatedly
	Teach rules step-by-step
	Post rules on wall
	Teach unwritten rules
	Explain inappropriate behavior
	Enroll in social skills group
	Use story boards
	Model appropriate social behavior
	Prompt child to watch peers' social behavior
	Teach through role-playing
Isolates self from peers	Create opportunities for fun with others
	Encourage playing with peers
	Assign play buddy
	Allow child to help out in younger classroom
	Teach how to start, maintain, and end play
	Provide fun group experiences
	Seat child near other special-needs students
	Assign lunch buddy
	Drama class
Cannot read body language	Teacher or library helper during lunch/recess
	Teach each body language and its meaning
	Explain body language as it occurs
	Prompt to guess what body language means
	Story boards
	Movie therapy
	Social skills group
	Role play

Lacks empathy	Explain meaning of others' emotions
	Prompt to guess meaning of others' emotions
	Prompt child to ask how others feel
Lacks tact	Explain impact on others
	Prompt to guess impact on others
	Model appropriate tact
	Role play
	Social skills therapy
	Movie therapy
Misinterprets people's intentions	Explain others' intentions to child
	Prompt child to ask people about their intentions
	Teach social cues that tell about intentions
	Encourage avoiding negative assumptions

WHAT YOUR AD CHILD WANTS YOU TO KNOW

- I may overreact for no apparent reason, but usually I have a reason I just can't say yet.
- Just because I was able to control myself for several days does not mean I can today.
- I don't misbehave on purpose, and I am not trying to defy or annoy you.
- Don't expect me to be smart in every subject just because I have a great vocabulary.
- Please don't tell me to "work it out" with my classmates, I have no idea how to do that.
- I love to talk and do not know when to stop. Gently remind me to "hold that thought."
- I am at my best when every day goes predictably. Please try to have a routine in class.
- Please warn me in advance of upcoming changes since I do not cope well with change.
- Keep a close eye on me in group activities because I do not do well in groups.
- I am at risk for trouble when I have unstructured time. Please help me find things to do.
- I learn and understand best with visual materials. I like charts, pictures, and schedules.

- I have to be told in each setting how to behave even if it is similar to other settings.
- I like to be asked or suggested rather than rigidly forced to do something.
- Please give me a place to go to if I feel like I am getting out of control.
- I respond best to calm and patient authority figures.
- I can complete things best if you tell me only one step at a time.
- When I talk about the same thing over and over please gently suggest I talk about it later.
- I am overly sensitive to criticism and will overreact to being told I am wrong.
- I will stop my misbehavior more if you redirect me instead of criticizing me.
- I am at risk for trouble with transitions and will do better if you help me create a routine.
- I can follow directions better if you tell me one at a time.
- I understand explanations and instructions better when they are short and simple.
- Sounds, lights, smells, textures, and touch may upset me greatly, and I have to get away.
- I am not good at games or ball, and I may refuse to play because I am embarrassed.
- I do my best when the setting is quiet, calm, and not too stimulating.
- I respond well to visual cues (e.g., pointing to your ear for me to listen).
- I am slow to respond if you ask me a question so please give me time to answer.
- My brain does not work well if I am interrupted. I usually insist on starting all over again.

- Please do not insist that I look you in the eye. I am very uncomfortable with eye contact.
- When I lose control over my anger please send me to my quiet place to calm down.
- I just can't ignore the teasing, so please help me find nice children to play with.
- I don't understand jokes or sarcasm so you might have to explain them to me.
- I follow instructions better when they are repeated several times.
- Even though nothing anyone does can cure me, I need your support every day all year.

TEACHER INFORMATION LIST

Use this list to fill in the blanks with the unique characteristics about your child. This list can be given to teachers, coaches, baby-sitters, relatives, and any other adults caring for your child.

Child's Name: Age: Grade:

Rewards that work	Organizational skills requiring help
Social activities he does well with	Social activities he has trouble with
Special interests	Sensory sensitivities
Words that inspire	Words that cause negative reactions

Problematic transitions	Changes he must be told about
Motor skills strengths	Motor skills difficulties
Behaviors he insists on doing	Other

BEHAVIOR CHARTS

Behavior Bubble

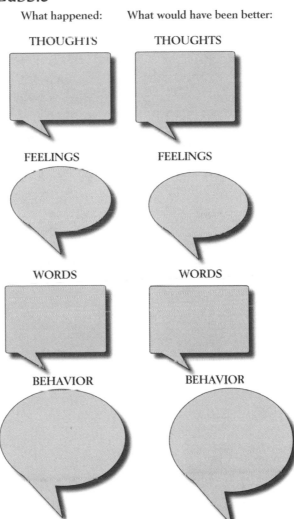

What happened: What would have been better:

THOUGHTS   THOUGHTS

FEELINGS   FEELINGS

WORDS   WORDS

BEHAVIOR   BEHAVIOR

Behavior Chart

List behaviors your child does in the Behavior column. In the Goal column write if you would like the behavior to increase or decrease. Select which behavior modification technique you will use to increase or decrease the behavior; positive reinforcement, negative reinforcement, positive punishment, or negative punishment. In the Consequence column write what will happen if your child does the specific behavior. See page 216 for a description on how to use these techniques.

Behavior	Goal	Technique	Consequence

Functional Behavior Analysis

See page 223 to learn how to use this chart for specific behavior problems your child displays.

Behavior	
Location	
Intensity	
Frequency	
Duration	
Antecedents	
Consequences	
Course	
Preventing the antecedents	
Changing the consequence	
Modifying the environment	
Teaching appropriate behavior	
Prompting appropriate behavior	
Rewarding appropriate behavior	

RECOMMENDED READING AND RESOURCES

Chapter 1: The ABCs of Asperger's Disorder
Websites with helpful information for those beginning their journey with AD

- www.asperger.org
- www.tonyattwood.com.au/
- www.aspergersyndrome.org
- www.aane.autistics.org
- www.nas.org.uk
- www.aspennj.org
- www.aspergerssyndrome.org
- www.jpk.com

Chapter 2: Getting Your Child Evaluated

- American Psychiatric Association. *Diagnostic and Statistical Manual of Mental Disorders IV-TR.* Washington, D.C.: American Psychiatric Association. 2000.

  Manual of mental disorders with diagnostic criteria and descriptions. Written for trained mental health professionals.

- Patricia Romoanowski Bashe, M.S. Ed., and Barbara L. Kirby. *Oasis Guide to Asperger's Syndrome.* New York: Crown Publishers. 2001, 2005.

  Written by two parents who raised children with AD, one of whom is an educational therapist, this book is like having the authors give you a pep talk.

Chapter 3: Coexisting Disorders

- American Psychiatric Association. *Diagnostic and Statistical Manual of Mental Disorders IV-TR*. Washington, D.C.: American Psychiatric Association. 2000.

    Manual of mental disorders with diagnostic criteria and descriptions. Written for trained mental health professionals.

- Ashley, Susan. *The ADD & ADHD Answer Book: The Top 275 Questions Parents Ask*. Naperville, Illinois: Sourcebooks, Inc. 2005.

    Comprehensive book about ADD and ADHD with useful tips to manage problems also commonly seen in children with AD.

- Comings, D. *Tourette's Syndrome and Human Behavior*. Duarte, California: Hope Press. 1990.

    Authoritative textbook on Tourette's.

- Learning Disability Online website: www.ldonline.com

    Information on learning disabilities.

- Ashley Psychology Center: www.ashleypsychology.com

    Website with useful information about various childhood psychological disorders.

Chapter 4: Social Skills

- Schab, L. *The You & Me Workbook: A Book That Teaches Social Skills and Social Awareness*. Plainview, New York: Childswork/Childsplay. 2001.

    Fun and quick exercises for children and preteens to increase social skills. Easy for parents and teachers to use.

- Jackson, N., Jackson, D. and Monroe, C. *Skill Lessons & Activities: Getting Along with Others, Teaching Social Effectiveness to Children*. Champaign, Illinois: Research Press. 1983.

    Lesson plans for teachers or group therapists to use to teach social skills.

- Kincher, J. *Psychology for Kids: 40 Fun Tests That Help You Learn about Yourself.* Minneapolis, Minnesota: Free Spirit Publishing, Inc. 1995.

    Fun exercises for children and teens to increase self-awareness. Parents can give this book to their child to read and use at his leisure.

- Zimmerman, T. and Shapiro L. *Sometimes I Feel Like I Don't Have Friends (But Not So Much Anymore): A Self-Esteem Book to Help Children Improve Their Social Skills.* King of Prussia, Pennsylvania: The Center for Applied Psychology, Inc. 1996.

    Fun short story for parents or teachers to read to children or simply give the book to the child to read on his own.

- Berg, B. *The Social Skills Workbook: Exercises to Improve Social Skills.* Dayton, Ohio: Cognitive Therapeutics. 1990.

    Exercises to be used in group setting by therapists or teachers to teach social skills.

- Berg. B. *The Anger Control Workbook: Exercises to Develop Anger Control Skills.* Dayton, Ohio: Cognitive Therapeutics. 1990.

    Exercises to be used with older children and teens to teach anger recognition and anger-management skills. Can be used independently by a motivated teen.

- Mannix, D. *Social Skills Activities for Special Children.* West Nyack, New York: Prentice Hall: 1993.

    Fun exercises for children to do in class, in group therapy, or at home with parents.

- American Girl Library. *The Care and Keeping of Friends.* Middleton, Wisconsin: Pleasant Company Publications. 1996.

    Fun book for girls to read to improve friendship skills.

- American Girl Library. *Oops! The Manners Guide for Girls.* Middleton, Wisconsin: Pleasant Company Publications. 1997.

    Fun, colorful book for girls to read alone or with their parent.

- Delmege, S. *Girl Friends: How to Be Friends Forever.* New York: Scholastic, Inc. 2002.

   Fun book to help children and teen girls learn how to be a good friend. Can be read alone or with a parent.
- Carlson, N. *How to Lose All Your Friends.* New York: Viking. 1994.

   By far the most requested book by children to have read to them in social skills therapy. A funny book that teaches children why they lose friends.
- Freedman, J. *Easing the Teasing. Helping Your Child Cope with Name-Calling, Ridicule and Verbal Bullying.* Chicago, Illinois: Contemporary Books. 2002.

   Describes a variety of useful techniques for parents to teach their child how to cope with teasing.
- Department of Education. http://www.ed.gov/about/offices/list/ocr/sexharassresources.html

   Website with information about schools' responsibilities in addressing students who are harassed.
- Rivannamusic. www.rivannamusic.com

   Website with music CDs teaching young children social skills through songs. Includes downloadable visual cues and lyrics for each social skill.
- Carnegie, Dale. *How to Win Friends & Influence People* (1936) New York: Pocket Books.

   Over 15 million copies of this book have been sold. Written to teach adults how to use social skills to become more likeable and improve relationships. Parents and adults with AD alike will greatly benefit from reading this book.
- Picture Communication Symbols.
   Mayer-Johnson LLC; P.O. Box 1579; Solana Beach, CA 92075
   Phone: 858-550-0084; Fax: 858-550-0449
   Email: mayerj@mayer-johnson.com
   Website: www.mayer-johnson.com

Chapter 5: Thinking Patterns

- Bogdashina, Olga. *Theory of Mind and the Triad of Perspectives on Autism and Asperger Syndrome.* London: Jessica Kingsley Publishers. 2005.

  Book to increase understanding of Theory of Mind.

- Michelle Garcia Winner. *Thinking About You, Thinking About Me: Philosophy and Strategies for Facilitating the Development of Perspective Taking for Students with Social Cognitive Deficits.* Michelle Garcia Winner. 2003.

  Book for parents and teachers to increase children's ability to use Theory of Mind.

- Baron-Cohen, Simon. *Mindblindness: An Essay on Autism and Theory of Mind.* Cambridge: The MIT Press. 1997.

  Book to increase understanding of Theory of Mind.

Chapter 6: Emotional Intelligence

- www.ccoder.com/GainingFace

  Website that helps children learn about feelings and how to read people's expressions.

- www.spectrumconnections.com/store.php

  Website to purchase music therapy videos and CDs to teach children about emotions.

- Shapiro, L. *How to Raise a Child with a High EQ: A Parents' Guide to Emotional Intelligence.* New York: Perennial Currents. 1998.

  Excellent book for parents that focuses on the emotional life of children.

- Trower, T. *The Self-Control Patrol Workbook: Exercises for Anger Management.* Plainview, New York: Childswork/Childsplay. 1995.

  Fun and quick one-page exercises for children and preteens to help increase awareness of anger and how to gain control over it. Can be used by parents, teachers, youth group and scout lead-ers, or even read by teens alone.

- Vernon, Ann. *Thinking, Feeling, Behaving: An Emotional Education Curriculum for Adolescents*. Champaign, Illinois: Research Press. 1989.

  Exercises and topics for discussion with pre-teen and teens. Can be used by parents, teachers, youth group and scout leaders, or even read by teens alone.

- Greenspan, S. *The Essential Partnership: How Parents can Meet the Emotional Challenges of Infancy and Childhood*. New York: Viking. 1989.

  An essential book for parents to learn psychological techniques to build a strong emotional relationship with their child.

- Schab, L. *The Anger Solution Workbook*. Plainview, New York: Childswork/Childsplay. 2001.

  Fun and quick exercises for children and teens to learn anger-management skills. Can be used with teacher, parents, or alone by child.

- Goleman, Daniel. *Emotional Intelligence: Why it can matter more than IQ*. New York: Bantam Books. 1995.

  Groundbreaking book to teach parents what emotional intelligence is and why it is so important to develop in yourself and your child. Adults with AD would also greatly benefit from this book.

Chapter 7: Special Interests, Routines, and Play

- Child's Work Child's Play, www.childswork.com

  Website to purchase games for special needs children.

Chapter 8: Language, Motor Skills, and Sensory Sensitivity

- American Occupational Therapy Association, www.aota.org
- American Speech-Language Hearing Association, www.asha.org

Chapter 9: Succeeding in School

- Office of Special Education Programs: www.ed.gov
  Information about special education.
- Council for Exceptional Children: www.cec.sped.org
  Information about special education including IDEA.
- No Child Left Behind, U.S. Department of Education: www.ed.gov
  Information about No Child Left Behind Act.
- Section 504, U.S. Department of Education: www.ed.gov
  Information about Section 504.
- FAQ about Special Education: www.wrightslaw.com
  Comprehensive website written specifically for parents addressing all areas of special education.
- Educational Resources Information Center: www.eric.ed.gov
  Information about special education.
- Educational Testing Service: www.ets.org
  Website describes necessary procedures for obtaining accommodations for college entrance examinations.
- Bridges 4 Kids: www.Bridges4kids.org
  Website with useful tips for assisting AD students in school.
- Baker, Linda J., and Welkowitz, Lawrence A. Editors. *Asperger's Syndrome: Intervening in Schools, Clinics and Communities.* Mahwah, New Jersey: Lawrence Erlbaum Associates, Publishers. 2005.
  Tips on helping students with AD succeed in school.

Chapter 10: Improving Behavior

- Kaplan, Joseph. *Kid Mod: Empowering Children and Youth Through Instructions in the Use of Reinforcement Principles.* Austin, Texas: Pro-Ed. 1996.
  Fun exercises for children and preteens to help them increase awareness of their choices, behavior, and consequences. Can be used by parents, teachers, and youth group and scout leaders.

- Garber, S., Garber, M., and Spizman, R. *Good Behavior: Over 1200 Sensible Solutions to Your Child's Problems from Birth to Age Twelve.* New York: Villard Books. 1987.

  Easy-to-use reference book of solutions for the most common behavior problems.
- Dinkmeyer, D., McKay, G., and Dinkmeyer, D. *The Parent's Handbook: STEP: Systematic Training for Effective Parenting.* Circle Pines, Minnesota: American Guidance Service. 1997.

  One of my favorite books on the basic techniques every parent should use.
- Eimers, R. and Aitchison, R. *Effective Parents Responsible Children: A Guide to Confident Parenting.* New York: McGraw-Hill Book Company. 1977.

  Another of my favorite books on parenting. Teaches parents how to use the behavior-modification techniques psychologists use.
- Gordon, T. *P.E.T.: Parent Effectiveness Training: The Proven Program for Raising Responsible Children.* New York: Three Rivers Press. 2000.

  A classic book on parenting and one of the all-time best, in print since 1970. Teaches verbal skills to help parents talk and listen to their child and learn to understand one another, negotiate, and resolve conflicts.

Chapter 11: Self-Esteem

- Kaufman, G., Raphael, L., and Espelan, P. *Stick up for Yourself: Every Kid's Guide to Personal Power and Self-Esteem.* Minneapolis, Minnesota: Free Spirit Publishing. 1999.

  Helpful guide for children who are teased to read either alone or with parents.

- Sharpiro, L. *Sometimes I Drive My Mom Crazy, But I Know She's Crazy About Me: A Self-Esteem Book for ADHD Children.* Plainview, New York: Childswork/Childsplay. 1995.
  Fun story every child with ADD or ADHD should read either alone or with their parents.

Chapter 12: Growing up with Asperger's

- University students with autism and Asperger's Syndrome: http://www.users.dircon.co.uk./~cns/index.html
- National Autistic Society: www.nas.org.uk
  Website based in the United Kingdom with useful information on various aspects for children and adults with AD.
- Families of Adults Afflicted with Asperger's Syndrome: www.faaas.org
  Website with useful information for adults with AD and their families.
- Fast, Yvona. *Employment for Individuals with Asperger's Syndrome or Non-Verbal Learning Disability.* London: Jessica Kingsley Publishers. London. 2004.
  Book for adults to help with succeeding in the workforce.
- Wrong Planet: www.wrongplanet.net
  Website for adults with AD.
- Lars Perner, Ph.D.: www.larsperner.com
  Website written by a college professor with AD. Helpful tools for college students with AD.
- Hénault, Isabelle. *Asperger's Syndrome and Sexuality: From Adolescence through Adulthood.* London: Jessica Kingsley Publishers. 2005.
  Book to help parents and teens, as well as adults, approach sexuality in healthy ways.

Index

About the Author

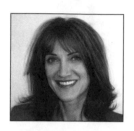 Susan Ashley, Ph.D., is the founder and director of Ashley Children's Psychology Center. Her training at UCLA Neuropsychiatric Institute, UCLA Infant and Child Studies laboratory, UCLA Child Care Center, San Fernando Valley Child Guidance Clinic and Camarillo State Hospital Child and Adolescent Units makes Dr. Ashley highly skilled in treating the most challenging children and adolescents.